Comparative National Policies on Health Care

POLITICAL SCIENCE AND PUBLIC ADMINISTRATION
A Program of Textbooks and Monographs

Executive Editors

KENNETH FRIEDMAN
Department of Political Science
Purdue University
West Lafayette, Indiana

NICHOLAS L. HENRY
Center for Public Affairs
Arizona State University
Tempe, Arizona

Further volumes in preparation

Developmental Editor
Comparative National Policies on Health Care

RALPH A. STRAETZ
Department of Politics
Political Science and Health Policy
New York University
New York, N. Y.

Comparative National Policies on Health Care

Milton I. Roemer

School of Public Health
University of California
Los Angeles, California

MARCEL DEKKER, INC.   New York and Basel

Library of Congress Cataloging in Publication Data

Roemer, Milton Irwin, 1916-
   Comparative national policies on health care.

   (Political science and public administration ; 2)
   Includes bibliographies and index.
   1. Medical policy. I. Title. II. Series.
RA393.R59   362.1'04'2   76-50384
ISBN 0-8247-6567-2

MARCEL DEKKER, INC.

270 Madison Avenue, New York, New York 10016

Current printing (last digit):
10 9 8 7 6 5 4 3 2

PRINTED IN THE UNITED STATES OF AMERICA

PREFACE

This book aims to provide an overview of health care systems throughout the world and the policies that guide them. Inevitably it has been written from the perspective of an American public health physician, but every effort has been made to view the various components of the subject with neutrality and objectivity. By noting the many and diverse ways that different nations cope with a health problem, the reader may gain some perspective on the methods employed in his own country with respect to corresponding problems.

In order to render so large a subject manageable, two types of simplification have been applied. Health care systems have been simplified by analyzing them in accordance with certain major components:

> economic support of health services
> health manpower resources
> health care facilities
> patterns of delivering medical care
> patterns of delivering preventive services
> regulation of health care
> methods of health administration and planning

There are doubtless other ways of examining and describing health service systems, but these seven attributes have been found useful for clarifying the main features. Within each component there are many details, and only the more important of these will be considered.

The second form of simplification has been with respect to the wide range of countries of the world. No two nations are exactly alike, and no two health care systems in the approximate 150 countries of the world are precisely the same. It is feasible, however, to cluster nations into a small number of "types." To do this, a classification has been used that may not be logically "pure," but which attempts to take account of both political and economic realities in the world today. Thus, countries are considered as falling under one or another of the following main types:

free enterprise
welfare states
underdeveloped
transitional
socialist

Placing a country in one or another of these five categories has been based on its *predominant* characteristics. To some extent every nation contains features which are found in different degrees in almost all other nations. However, those characteristics of the country's political structure and level of economic development which seem to have the greatest influence on its health care system are the basis of the classification. In the discussion of each feature of the health care system, an effort has been made to offer illustrations from more than one country of each of the five types.

In order to present this account in an easy, discursive style, I have not followed the usual practice of scholarly annotation. Instead, there appears at the end of each chapter a list of references that give a great deal of further information on the subjects discussed. Many citations contain material relevant to more than one chapter.

A world review of this scope is bound to be somewhat superficial. However, the very purpose of this book has been to achieve a kind of panorama view of national health care systems, rather than in-depth probing of any one feature or any one country. In the 330-plus citations of the "Readings," one will find numerous reports of a more specialized character.

The preparation of this book has been an outgrowth of a teaching project on "International Health," sponsored by the Association of American Medical Colleges. To Dr. Emanuel Suter of the AAMC and several colleagues on the Association's International Program Advisory Committee, I am indebted for many stimulating discussions and helpful suggestions. I am especially grateful to Dr. Suter for his encouragement to publish this volume, in supplementation of the self-instructional text for medical students coming from his project. I am very grateful also to Dr. Ray Elling for access to his comprehensive bibliographic materials on comparative health care systems.

This book is also an outgrowth of the author's work—usually as a foreign consultant—in some forty-five countries of all five conceptual types, from 1950 to the present. The foreign observer usually acquires an oversimplified impression of a nation's attributes. Although the defects of such perception are obvious, one advantage is that the observer sees the national picture in broad outline, often in a configuration not seen by those who live daily and closely with a country's problems.

The foreign observer may also have the benefit of meeting key national health leaders, crucial decision-makers of a level he may seldom encounter in his native land. Since time is often limited, the observer may be in a position to pick up a great deal of information offered in brief conversations. I have been the fortunate beneficiary of many such informative meetings, and I am enormously indebted to the health system leaders that I have met. I hope that the interpretations of what they taught me, offered in these pages, give a reasonably accurate picture of the many ways that mankind has mobilized its resources for the health care of populations.

Milton I. Roemer, M.D.

CONTENTS

1

INTRODUCTION AND OVERVIEW
OF HEALTH SERVICE SYSTEMS

In a sense, the world may be regarded as a great laboratory in which many experiments are being conducted on different methods of organizing and providing health service. If we can study these diverse experiments objectively, we can learn a lot about both the determinants and the effects of varying health care systems. To lead into this study we will consider first the underlying circumstances of different approaches to providing health care—the historical, economic, political, cultural, and other factors involved. We will then attempt to characterize the countries of the world according to the main types of health care system in them: the predominantly free enterprise model, the welfare states, the different levels of developing and transitional countries, and the socialist nations. Then, in this introductory chapter, we will consider the general scope of the subjects to follow, that is, the dimensions along which health care systems may be analyzed.

Determinants of Health Care Systems

Any analysis of the determinants of a social situation is necessarily artificial, for we are forced to abstract certain causative influences as if they operated independently. In fact, the whole process of social development is a complex mixture of many different influences that interplay among one another as well as upon the phenomenon we are studying, which is health services.

Still, to analyze these complicated dynamics, we have to dissect them into separate pathways. So, for the sake of clarification, we can consider the determinants of health care systems under four main categories: (a) historical determinants, (b) economic levels, (c) political policies, and (d) other cultural influences. We cannot be comprehensive about any of these determinants, but perhaps some examples under each category will indicate the great extent to which a health care system is the product of social influences of several types.

Historical Background

It has been said that those who do not know the past are condemned to repeat it, and this is as true of developments in the health services as of anything else. The medical student may learn to understand the circulation of the blood without knowing about William Harvey's *De Motu Cordis,* which in 1628 refuted the erroneous teachings of Galen that had for centuries been accepted as correct. He is not so likely, however, to understand the meaning and implications of America's Blue Cross hospitalization plans without having some knowledge of the early origins of the health insurance movement in Europe. Moreover, the very rise of health insurance as a method for financing medical care must be traced to much larger events in the development of European civilization. Let us consider some examples of these historical forces.

The United States emerged as an independent nation after a revolution against the British crown starting in 1776. A crucial aspect of the ideology of that American Revolution was opposition to centralized authority, whether it was represented by a distant monarch in London or any other authority. The Constitution that emerged from such a revolution naturally incorporated all sorts of checks and balances among the executive, legislative, and judicial branches of the central government. It also established the sovereignty of the component states, originally thirteen British colonies, in most matters of government, reserving for the states all responsibilities not specifically assigned to the federal government, such as the conduct of foreign relations or the regulation of interstate commerce. Among the many matters remaining under the authority of the states was the protection of health.

Thus, the licensing of doctors, the operation of public health programs, the planning of hospital construction, and countless other aspects of health care are still, 200 years after the nation's birth, state responsibilities. Insofar as the whole socioeconomic situation has changed, yielding greater powers of money raising (taxation) in the national government, financial support for health purposes is furnished largely through federal grants-in-aid to the states. Certain standards may be imposed for the allocation of these grants, but the final decisions on the use of federal grant money rest with the state governments. These attributes of the everyday operation of our health care system must obviously be traced to the American Revolution.

Consider also the French Revolution of 1789. The rebellion was not only against the monarchy but also its allies—the great feudal landowners and the Catholic church. The church, among other things, owned and operated most hospitals in France at the time. When a parliamentary National Assembly was set up in the first French republic, it was natural that the hospitals should be transferred to secular authorities. France was divided eventually into about ninety *départements* or provinces, each of which was assigned responsibility for the church hospitals in its borders. Under the Napoleonic laws promulgated after the revolution, rather strong central controls were established; a centrally appointed prefect or governor was delegated the authority in each department. Among other things, he was responsible for public properties, including the hospitals. The prefect appointed a health officer to whom he assigned these responsibilities, with advice from an elected council of citizens who represented the several *arrondissements* in the department. To this day, the French public hospitals are operated by the departmental governments under laws and regulations issued by the national government—all an outgrowth of the French Revolution.

In earlier periods, the hospitals in Europe had been founded largely by the Christian church. Christianity taught pity for and kindness to the poor and the sick; hospitals were a practical way of implementing this philosophy. It was natural that at first, in the early Middle Ages, these facilities should extend their charity to the aged and destitute as well as the sick. The advancement of science was necessary before "hostels" could evolve into hospitals run specifically for the sick. To staff the hospitals there were holy sisters or nuns who were, of course, the precursors of the modern nurse. They worked without compensation, since they were serving the Lord; their objective was to heal the soul of the patient, as much as his body, through frequent daily prayers.

It took the practical demands of the British war in the Russian Crimea (1853-1856) to inspire an English woman, Florence Nightingale, to organize teams of young women unconnected with any church to go overseas and nurse the wounded soldiers. On her return, realizing the need for proper skills to nurse the sick effectively, Miss Nightingale founded in 1860 the first formal school of nursing at St. Thomas' Hospital in London. Perhaps this professional discipline would have developed eventually anyway, but surely the dramatic circumstances of the Crimean War had much to do with the origins of modern nursing at that time and place. And it is equally certain that the great expansion of hospitals in the late nineteenth century, an expansion associated with the discovery of pathogenic bacteria and the benefits of antisepsis and asepsis, laid the groundwork for nursing's rapid growth.

Consider the whole development of cities as an aspect of the industrial revolution. Crowded housing around factories laid the basis for the spread of infectious disease, both through person-to-person contacts and through media such as food and water. Even ancient Rome had recognized the necessity of a system of public sewage disposal, with its *cloaca maxima.* Dr. John Snow traced the cholera epidemic in London in 1854 to polluted wells long before the discovery of the pathogenic organism. Such epidemics made clear the need for sanitary public water supply systems for urban populations. Even today the best developed safe water systems everywhere in the world are found in the largest cities, which are, or course, the result principally of industrialization.

The Industrial Revolution of the eighteenth and nineteenth centuries also had many other implications for health care systems. Concentrations of low-paid workers naturally gave rise to cooperative mutual aid societies, which in turn led to social insurance for health care. The political consequences of such concentrations of workers were equally relevant with the rise of Socialist parties and the actions of Germany's conservative Chancellor Bismarck to "steal their thunder" with the first social insurance laws in the 1880s. Industrialization also led to accidents from hazardous machinery, generating first the employer's liability laws and then the industrial injury compensation acts that provide socially insured medical care for the worker injured on the job.

Consider the influence of colonialism on the organization of health services in the dependent lands of Africa and Asia. Although the first concern of the European colonial powers was to protect their own overseas armies and settlers, eventually the effective exploitation of foreign natural resources required a minimum framework of public health and medical services. The British-controlled Indian Medical Service (IMS), for example, established a hierarchy of authority to operate hospitals and dispensaries and to maintain some regulation over urban sanitation in the nineteenth century. The semimilitary style of the IMS was an outgrowth of the colonial government, and after India's emancipation in 1947 it inevitably influenced the framework of the new Indian Ministry of Health. As in the IMS, all doctors in modern India's government health service are full-time civil servants. This is not the case, however, in Latin American countries, where the health ministries have developed in recent times without colonial antecedents.

In Africa the colonial authorities could not attract many doctors or nurses from Europe. The only practical solution to the staffing of hospitals was to train native men—to a lesser extent, women—to assist in the medical work. Hence, the African "dresser" was taught by apprenticeship and became the most numerous type of health worker in these colonies. When liberation of most African countries occurred after World War II, the major manpower base of the new health service systems was the relatively large corps of dressers and other medical assistants. Now, however, these personnel are given more systematic training, and local medical schools have been established. The current concept of auxiliary health manpower in Africa is clearly an outgrowth of nineteenth century colonialism.

History is not only a matter of the distant past but constitutes the whole sequence of events up to the present moment. Consider such recent history as the Great Depression of the 1930s, the Cuban Revolution of 1959, or the sudden elevation of the world price of oil in the 1970s. One can identify all sorts of results of the impact of such historical events on the shape of health care systems. The Depression gave rise to the Social Security Act in the United States in 1935, and eventually it resulted in Medicare for the aged in 1965. The Cuban Revolution led not only to the total reorganization of health services in that country but had impacts on health planning throughout Latin America. And the rise in oil prices has, among many other effects, led to a great expansion of hospitals and health centers in Iran, Saudi Arabia, and other oil-producing nations. It has meant also an energy crisis in the United States that has caused an invigoration of the coal mining industry. This, in turn, has rejuvenated health services for coal miners and their families through a large welfare fund that only a few years before was reducing its health program.

These are perhaps enough examples of the impact of historical events on health care systems. Indeed, every component of every nation's efforts to provide health service has its history which, if traced, will invariably show influences from social events far outside the boundaries of medicine or public health.

Economic Levels

History is a composite of developments in the economic, political, and other cultural sectors of society. We may consider separately, nevertheless, how current economic levels throughout the world, or even different degrees of economic development within one country, influence the health care system.

Most fundamentally, the economic level of a country determines largely, although not entirely, its ability to generate resources for the health care of its population. For example, training of doctors is costly whether it is done by governmental or private educational institutions. In fact, the high cost of modern medical education has made the great majority of medical schools in nearly all countries dependent on government for their support. This is true whether the schools and their parent universities are sponsored entirely by government, or sponsored by private bodies and subsidized with public grants. The same applies only in lesser degree to schools for training dentists, pharmacists, technicians, and other health personnel. (Nursing schools attached to hospitals can recover some of their costs by getting uncompensated labor from the nursing students, but this very fact may reduce their educational effectiveness and has led in many countries to separation of nursing schools from the hospitals.)

Because of the high costs of training health manpower, the rate of output of such manpower is largely dependent on a country's economic strength. In affluent America, there is one medical school for about every 1.8 million persons; in impoverished Ethiopia, the first medical school was recently developed to prepare doctors for its over 25 million people. Other noneconomic factors also play a part, as illustrated by the nine medical schools that train doctors for Australia's population of only 13 million with two more schools being planned. Each school is regarded as a regional center for medical services as well as for training. Similarly, immediately after its revolution in 1959, Cuba developed three medical schools for its population of 9 million when only one had existed for the previous fifty years.

The output of doctors and other health personnel is likewise related to a country's economic capacity to support their work. In Latin America, for example, the supply of physicians and dentists in relation to population has been steadily rising in step with the increased capacity of social insurance programs to finance medical services. On the other hand, some countries may for various reasons train more doctors, nurses, or other medical personnel than they can economically sustain; as a result, a great deal of outmigration of recent graduates occurs. This was previously true of Austria, where Viennese medical schools turned out many more graduates than the country could absorb. Since about 1950 it has been true of the Philippines, where an unusually high proportion of privately owned medical schools produce several thousand graduates each year. Because the cities are economically saturated and most of the young doctors do not wish to face the hardship and low earnings of a rural location, over half of them emigrate, mainly to the United States. This "brain drain" from a poor country to a rich one only aggravates larger economic inequalities, and it is generating plans for corrective legislation.

The dependence of health manpower output on future earning capacity is illustrated by the field of podiatry in Australia. This type of health service has not been covered by that country's health insurance legislation. As a result, the demand for foot care is not great, and the average earnings of podiatrists are not very high. Therefore, more than threequarters of Australia's podiatrists, in sharp contrast to the United States, are women, whose income expectations have not been as high as men's. Pharmacists in Australia, on the other hand, are found in the exceptionally high ratio of about one per 1,000 of population (the U.S. ratio is 1:1600), nearly all of whom are men. This obviously is related to Australia's Pharmaceutical Benefits Act, which since 1950 has publically supported the cost of most drugs prescribed for the total population.

The correlation of hospitals and other health care facilities with a nation's wealth is equally clear. Haiti is an extremely poor island country where a total of about 3,500 hospital beds are available to serve the population of 5 million— or less than 0.75 beds per 1,000. Not far away is Canada with not only much greater wealth but with a national program of social insurance for hospital care; it cannot be surprising that Canada has about 10.0 beds per 1,000 of its population or more than thirteen times as many as Haiti proportionately. Some countries may, indeed, build more hospital beds than would be required with prudent economic planning, whereas others do not begin to meet their needs. In any event, economic resources are the basic determinant.

Not only the quantities of health care resources but the ways they are used in the health care system may be largely influenced by economic levels. In a wealthy nation with a robust free-market economy, a great deal of the time of physicians, dentists, pharmacists, optometrists, and others is typically devoted to private practice, that is, the sale of personal health services on a fee basis. The United States is the illustration of this pattern par excellence, and the pattern is seen even in a country such as France, where the vast majority of the population are covered by social insurance for medical care. The French social insurance program helps the patient pay most of his medical costs, but the doctor still remains a small private businessman, collecting fees for each unit of service.

On the other hand, in a Latin American country such as Ecuador, the great majority of doctors cannot make a satisfactory income in purely private practice. Insofar as possible, they take salaried positions, usually four or six hours a day, in the social security system, the ministry of health, the armed forces, private industries, or other organized health programs. The balance of their time will be devoted to private patients, but there simply are not enough people who can afford to pay private medical fees to support a greater volume of private practice. Only a few docotrs devote all their time to private practice.

Market dynamics affect the prices of medical care in capitalist economies. In prosperous times and places, medical or dental fees tend to be higher than in periods of depression or in poorer countries. Even at one time and place, in our American open-market setting, the doctor may charge a higher fee to a wealthy patient than to a poor one. Although this sliding scale of fees is often justified in terms of an equity process applied by each doctor in order to serve the poor at lower prices, economists generally consider it a special application of the well-known entrepreneurial strategy of "charging what the traffic will bear."

In more affluent countries, public revenues can be used to pay doctors and hospitals to care for the poor at reasonable rates. These charges may be paid through special public assistance programs, with the poor being served in private facilities. In less prosperous countries, the poor are usually served—if at all—in public clinics. In such clinics the doctor works on a salary, which yields lower per-service costs. Either way, it is the economic level that largely determines the pattern of providing health care.

To a large extent a nation's wealth is dependent on its degree of industrialization, and this has multiple influences on health care patterns. The economically more developed countries are more urbanized, transportation and communication in them are better, and the people are more highly educated. These social conditions affect both the demand for medical services and the supply. A large proportion of rural people in a nation, as in India or Nigeria, means a lesser demand for scientific medicine as well as greater difficulties in providing it. Urban concentration generates its own health problems, but it also facilitates the application of both preventive and therapeutic measures to cope with them.

Since World War II, wide-ranging programs of foreign aid have developed through which the wealthier industrialized countries help the poorer, agricultural countries. Although many political motives may lie behind these programs, and although the financial aid is often less than the profits extracted by multinational corporations, foreign technical assistance can exert great influence on national health care systems. The several mechanisms of bilateral or truly international agency assistance will be considered later, but at the root of these activities lie the differences in economic development among countries. Foreign aid is a channel through which health science technologies and even systems of health care organization are transmitted across national borders.

The level of economic development of a country determines the extent to which it must depend on other countries for drugs, medical equipment, and even scientific knowledge. Few of the less developed countries have chemical industries to produce modern medications; they must typically import these at relatively high costs. Even if pills or capsules are locally produced, their ingredients are usually imported. One of the first actions of India after its independence was to develop with foreign aid its own plants for producing antibiotic drugs. The same occurred in China and Cuba after their social revolutions.

Research to produce new scientific knowledge requires a great investment in the education of scientists as well as the production of elaborate equipment. It is small wonder that most (although, of course, not all) scientific discoveries for the prevention and treatment of disease have come from the highly developed nations of Europe and North America. This is not to overlook the achievements of ancient Indian Ayurvedic medicine in finding the antihypertensive effects of *Rauwolfia serpentina* or of ancient Chinese healing in discovering the value of acupuncture anesthesia. But on the whole, the main body of modern scientific medicine and public health knowledge has come from the more industrialized countries. Fortunately, the ethics of science have led to the wide dissemination of this knowledge through world-wide publication and in other ways.

Finally, it has been found that even the *share* of a nation's resources devoted to health service depends on its wealth. The more affluent countries spend around 5 to 8 percent of their gross national product (GNP) on all health-related purposes, whereas in poorer countries the comparable figure is 2 to 4 percent. The developing countries have to spend so large a share of their available resources for essentials such as food and shelter that there is relatively less left for health service; the latter gets a smaller slice of a smaller economic pie.

Political Policies

Perhaps most prominent in determining the social system by which health services are supported, organized, and distributed in a country are its political policies. Although it is interwoven with economic and other factors and although it often even alters what might be the "natural" market operation of economic forces, the exercise of political power according to one or another ideology has pervasive impacts on the quantity and delivery patterns of health services in a country.

Examples are legion. Consider the War on Poverty in the United States of the 1960s. With enormous political problems, both domestically and internationally, with a real war in Vietnam, it seemed to make good political sense to wage an honorable war at home against the deterioration of the big city slums! Little was done to strike at the basic causes of poverty, but there were numerous programs to ameliorate its consequences—child care centers or Operation Headstart, poverty law clinics, and wherever there was an urban riot, usually with strong racial overtones, the construction of neighborhood health centers. The U.S. Office of Economic Opportunity, which administered these programs, was dismantled within ten years, but in different forms the community health centers remain.

Consider the origins of social insurance for hospitalization and then physicians' care in Canada over the last generation. The concepts had been discussed by the conventional political parties since 1919, but it took the victory of the semisocialist Cooperative Commonwealth Federation (CCF) party in Saskatchewan in 1944 to lead in 1947 to the first social insurance program for hospital care of a total provincial population. Within ten years, all of Canada adopted the same idea. Then the pioneering in the sphere of doctors' care remained again for Saskatchewan to do in 1962. Despite a traumatic doctors' strike to usher it in, by 1968 the Canadian national government passed a law to spread physicians' care insurance through all ten provinces.

In Southeast Asia, the British rulers of the Malay Peninsula had turned over authority after World War II to the conservative sultans, in spite of the sultans' well-known role as collaborators with the Japanese during the war. Quite understandably this led to a guerrilla warfare opposition movement based in the villages and rural areas. Unlike the French in Vietnam, the British armies over a four-year period effectively repressed this movement by 1952. But in the new Malaysian Parliament, the political question was raised: "After all this bloodshed in the countryside, must we not do something beneficial for the rural people?" Thus began the Malaysian Rural Health Services Scheme in 1953, a program bringing hundreds of health centers and greatly improved preventive and treatment services to millions of poor people.

Consider the impact of politics on health services in Latin America. From the first social security program for medical care in Chile in 1924 to the most recent one in Uruguay in 1958, the political maturation and demands of the urban workers, who voted in elections, required attention. Many economic purposes were likewise fulfilled, but it is hardly likely that these health programs, which provided greatly improved services in the main cities, would have been launched without the growing political importance of industrial workers. The political revolution in Cuba in 1959, as noted earlier, brought a total change in the health care system of that country—a system modeled largely on that of Cuba's Soviet supporters and advisers. And with the right-wing military coup in Santiago in 1973 not only were the leaders of the Chilean National Health Service eliminated (many being killed, jailed, or exiled), but the entire structure of the service was weakened while private medical practice was strengthened.

The development of health care systems in Europe has been in large part a story of the battle for votes in parliamentary democracies. The continuous extension of health benefits in social security programs has paralleled the growth of social democratic and labor parties. So politically popular have these programs been that, even under conservative parties, the changes have been minor for fear of losing votes. When the Tories regained power after the British Labour Party had launched the National Health Service in 1948, the only significant change they made was to raise the personal co-payment for prescribed drugs from one shilling (14 U.S. cents) to two. The revolutions in Eastern Europe after World War II led inevitably to adoption of the socialist model of health system developed in the Soviet Union (USSR) after World War I.

The conservative (Liberal Party) government of Australia from 1950 to 1972 made it in those years the only industrialized country, aside from the United States, to lack a mandatory social insurance system for general medical care. Instead, there was an elaborately complex system of subsidized voluntary insurance, with little if any controls over the private sector. But soon after the Labor Party was elected in late 1972, the law was changed to launch a health insurance system with universal population coverage and wider benefits. In late 1975, the Liberal Party was again returned to power, but the broad new health care system was too popular to dismantle, and changes were made only to give private agencies a role in the administration of the program.

Examples could be multiplied, but it is quite obvious that health service has become in every country a volatile political issue. Yet in the larger political scene, it is not a very critical issue involving power relations to the extent seen in policies on land ownership, industrial control, or foreign relations. Therefore, even under moderately liberal or even conservative political parties, changes are made in the health care system to attract political support. Aside perhaps from alienating a relatively small number of health professionals—and often not even these—modifications in the health care system do not greatly disturb important centers of power. Therefore, health programs are what some often call a convenient political football or, more accurately, the programs are highly sensitive to relatively small changes in the political balance of power.

Other Cultural Factors

Finally, one may identify various other cultural or environmental factors that have impacts on the health care system. Generally, they are not as pervasive as the historical, economic, or political influences just reviewed, but some examples may be cited.

In the sphere of religion, the influence of the Catholic church on the field of family planning and population control has been prominent. Emphasizing the sanctity of human life and regarding life to begin, according to papal teaching, at the moment of fertilization of the human ovum, Catholic leadership has been opposed until recently to aborting any pregnancy, even to save the life of the mother. (Papal teaching has changed, so that abortion to save the mother's life is now generally condoned.) Clearly related is the Catholic view of contraception by physical or chemical mechanisms as interference with the "natural law" of reproduction. The rhythm method of contraception, based on sexual abstinence during certain days of the menstrual cycle, is acceptable, although it is known to have a wide margin of failure. As a result, the heavily Catholic continent of Latin America has the highest birth rate in the world. This clearly affects the demands on health services—not to mention the broader problems of population pressure—and also has led to a very high incidence of traumatic self-induced abortions or abortions performed by nonmedical personnel.

The Christian faith has taught compassion for the poor which, as we have already noted, gave rise to hospitals in the Middle Ages. It was likewise responsible for the early origins of nursing. Teachings of both Christianity and Judaism about "love thy neighbor" and the so-called Protestant ethic of saving for the future provided a spiritual basis for cooperative societies that led eventually to the worldwide health insurance movement.

Both the Hindu and the Moslem faiths teach the subordinate and servile role of women; the wife is the property of her husband, and it is sacrilegious for her to be touched or even viewed, by another man. Although these ideas are changing, they still exert an influence on the organization of health services in India and in many Moslem countries. A woman is supposed to be medically attended by another woman, not by a male doctor or medical aide. Health centers in rural India are officially staffed by a woman doctor as well as a male doctor, although women are very difficult to recruit for this work. The married woman is supposed to spend most of her time at home, so as not to be seen or tempted by men on the streets. Circumcision of girls (surgical excision of the clitoris) is still practiced in many Moslem countries to reduce sexual temptation in women. These attitudes and practices surely inhibit the utilization of medical services by women in cultures following these religions.

The sacred cow, to outsiders, is a virtual symbol of the Hindu faith. Its influence on the nutritional level of the people of India has been profound. Cows consume grain and other foods, yet the beef they could provide may not be consumed. By an opposite logic, but with similar consequences, the pig is "unclean" and unacceptable as food in both the Jewish and Moslem faiths. Hinduism teaches the sanctity of all animal life, even that of the smallest insect. Malaria control programs require the destruction of mosquitoes, and it was only when the great leader, Mahatma Ghandi, developed the formulation that the spraying of DDT led to the killing of mosquitoes not by man but by a chemical were these preventive campaigns fully accepted in India.

The Chinese, having no such religious restrictions, have greatly improved their health levels in recent years by massive destruction of "the four pests"— flies, mosquitoes, rats, and bedbugs.

The social institution of the family has many influences on health care. Studies of adult hospitalization show it to be highest among people outside an intact family—the unmarried, the divorced, or the widowed. Adjusting for age level, of course, the adult without close family ties lacks protection in time of illness and is more likely to require the care of a hospital. The honoring of the aged in oriental cultures means that grandparents are usually cared for by their adult children. In the more mobile western societies aged parents are usually left on their own; to help them economically, old-age pension programs have been organized. And when old age makes people feeble or sick, care in an institution is the customary solution.

Community structure is part of the cultural environment, with influences on the health care system that are usually taken for granted. The concept of regionalization of hospital and ambulatory services that is being applied in almost all countries rests fundamentally on the ecology of large cities, small towns, and rural areas. To render medical services efficiently, use must be made of channels of communication and transportation developed in a region for many social and economic reasons outside the health field. City life may create special disease hazards, but it also makes possible the mobilization of resources to cope with the consequences.

These social influences—historical, economic, political, and cultural—are obviously intermeshed, constantly changing, and operating in different ways at different times and places. They combine to shape the character of the health service system one finds in each of the approximately 140 nations of the globe. Since the nation-state plays so crucial a role in world affairs and in the daily lives of individuals, it is helpful to examine the nations of the world and attempt to classify them into a number of basic types. Numerous systems of classification might be employed, but here we shall use an approach to shed special light on the patterns of health services.

National Types of Health Care System

Depending on the objective, the nations of the world have been classified in many ways. In the period of the Roman Empire, statesmen saw the sectors of the world that they controlled as "civilized," all the rest being "barbarian." With the rise of Christianity, the globe was divided between the realms of that faith and all the rest—the "pagans." In the nineteenth century, when competition for the control of the earth's resources was prominent, Europeans spoke of the "have" and "have-not" nations.

More recently, in the strategy to form a United Nations after World War II, political realists spoke of the "great powers" and the remainder of the smaller nations as "lesser powers." Later, when colonies were emancipated and the inequalities among people became extremely visible, demanding corrective actions, the fashion was to categorize countries as "underdeveloped" (later "developing") or "developed." As the Cold War of political conflict grew more intense in the 1950s and 1960s, leaders of Western Europe and North America spoke of the "free world"—all the rest being hidden behind an "iron curtain" (or a "bamboo" one) in totalitarian bondage. All these typologies are obviously a great oversimplification, designed to influence how people should think and act, ultimately to shape political decisions on war and peace.

Turning to our objective of learning about the various health care systems that have evolved and, of course, are still evolving in the world, we may consider still another classification. Since political ideologies and economic levels, as we have seen, are major determinants of health care systems, one can design a classification of countries formed along both of these dimensions—a conceptual blending that some scholars define as "political economy." We can categorize countries in terms of the political economy of their health care systems.

None of these types of health care system is absolutely pure anywhere, since in every nation there are special variants or subsystems, and the complexity is compounded by further changes every year, even every month. However, in terms of the *predominant* characteristics of the health care systems of different nations, we can identify five principal types: (a) free enterprise, (b) welfare state, (c) underdeveloped, (d) transitional, and (e) socialist. One must emphasize that countries subsumed under each of these types are in continual flux. Even at one time, moreover, there is a spectrum of gradations within each category. With these cautions, we will consider the main characteristics of these five types of health care system.

Free Enterprise Systems

The world is changing so rapidly that there hardly remains a country with a health care system in which free enterprise, once common, is the predominant

mode of operation. The closest, undoubtedly, is the United States, although
even here changes have been so numerous in recent decades that a better illustration would be the United States in 1940. Similarly, moving backward a decade
or two, one would find this type of system illustrated in Australia and perhaps in
the Union of South Africa.

The essential characteristics of the free enterprise system are the development and use of health care resources in a predominantly open market, with
minimum intervention of government or other mechanisms of control over demand, supply, or price. Health services, in the main, are bought and sold like
other commodities. Since social interventions in this process are minimal, the
distribution of services is dependent mainly on individual purchasing power.
Also, efforts to modify this process are put forth mainly through private and
local initiative; thus a multiplicity of programs may develop to organize the
financing and/or delivery of health services for certain persons or against certain
diseases. This yields a pluralism of organized subsystems that depend on local
strength and creativity. At the same time, multiple programs reflect differentials
in money and power and yield great discrepancies in access to health care. The
relationship of health services to health needs is extremely uneven. Because of
the unfettered freedom of action, great health achievements may be possible.
Those who, for one reason or another, are talented, ingenious, wealthy, or
powerful gain rich opportunities to use medical science, both as providers and
recipients. Others without these attributes may suffer greatly for their lack.

If this picture seems overdrawn or melodramatic today, it is only because
events of the last few decades have changed it everywhere. Political pressures
to change it have been generated by the very unevenness of outputs of the free
enterprise system, with its inequities in relation to health needs. All sorts of
organized health programs have arisen to interrupt the free flow of economic
market forces and local political autonomies. Yet, as we will see in subsequent
chapters, the vestiges of earlier conditions remain, just as the contours of early
automobiles reflected the lines of the horsedrawn buggy.

To cite just one example in the United States, many programs of voluntary
medical care insurance have developed in the last forty years. The financial support for most inpatient health service has been collectivized. The hospital and
the doctor, however, still remain predominantly private and free agents. They
receive, as before, fees for each service rendered, although the fees are paid by
an insurance organization rather than the individual patient. As the insurance
program matures, it may impose certain controls or constraints on the performance of the health care providers; it may limit the size of fees or monitor the
content of services. Eventually, some hospitals or doctors may become quite
markedly affected, but for many years, the attributes of former days will remain visible.

The very process of collectivizing financial support for health services in the free enterprise American setting has been applied in large part by private corporations. The largest enrollment in so-called "voluntary health insurance plans" is through commercial insurance companies, usually with stockholders and in business for profit. The profit motive, of course, may offer incentives for certain efficiencies but, at the same time, may lead to deceptions and other abuses, such as unjustified surgical operations.

Welfare State Systems

When pressures in the industrialized countries have reached a point at which responsibilities for assuring health services to *most* of the population in accordance with their needs have been assumed by government, the resultant system can be described as that of a "welfare state." Equalizing access to health service has nearly always been achieved by collectivizing financial support through various social insurance mechanisms, to be described in the next chapter. Yet much of the provision of health service, as in the free enterprise system, remains still in private hands, with a variety of measures applied by government to control the quality and costs. The very social visibility of the costs and their escalation with advancing technology and utilization rates create political pressures for increasing the scope of the controls.

In the main, the welfare state systems of health service are seen in western Europe. Because of European historical development, the pattern of delivery of in-hospital and out-of-hospital service tends to be very different from that in free enterprise America. Hospitals are mainly, although not entirely, institutions controlled by government, usually local units of government. All the personnel in them, including the doctors, are typically on salaries. Only the most highly trained and specialized physicians and surgeons are permitted to work in most hospitals. Outside of facilities in the community, the great majority of doctors are general practitioners. When one of their patients is referred for hospitalization, he typically becomes transferred to the responsibility of a hospital doctor.

This pattern is most usually found in Great Britain and the Scandinavian countries. Variations are found in Germany, France, Belgium, Holland, Greece, Italy, and Spain. In Germany and France, for example, a majority of patients are served in public (governmental) hospitals, where this pattern prevails, but a large fraction of patients use voluntary hospitals where independent specialists, based principally in separate community offices, treat their private patients. The smallest use of salaried hospital doctors is probably seen in Belgium where, although inpatients are treated only by qualified specialists (with some exceptions for maternity care), these specialists are typically paid by the social insurance on a private fee basis.

Preventive services tend to be provided through quite separate channels in the welfare states. Since public health authorities originated in the community battles against epidemic diseases of earlier centuries, they have continued to function quite separately from curative medicine. Even when the scope of public health agencies has been broadened to include promotion of the health of children or the early detection of chronic diseases in adults, these activities have been carried out quite independently of day-to-day medical care. The administration of the social insurance laws is usually, though not always, by ministries of labor or welfare, rather than ministries of health, whose focus remains largely preventive.

In other parts of the world industrialized countries, influenced by Europe and emulating its practices, have also adopted welfare state systems of health care. This is especially true of Japan, New Zealand, and more recently, of Australia. Social insurance in these countries has made financial access to medical care universal or nearly so, even though private practice of the health professions outside of hospitals is the general rule. In Japan, even for medical service within hospitals, private delivery patterns are highly prevalent.

Underdeveloped Country Systems

In the very poorest countries, which one may clearly describe as underdeveloped rather than developing, resources for modern health service are extremely deficient. (Every country is, however, "developing" and the concept of development must essentially be relative.) This is true of nearly all the countries of Africa and much of Asia, especially Indonesia, Burma, Afghanistan, and Nepal. In these countries, the vast majority of the population are quite outside the reach of modern medical care. Being only very slightly industrialized, the population is predominantly rural, illiterate, and impoverished, with all the concomitants of malnutrition and disease.

This large majority of people depend for most of their health care on primitive traditional healers located in the villages. Most minor illness goes entirely untreated, and the more severe disorders are typically brought to the attention of the village healers, who may be of various mystical or empirical types. Insofar as modern medical science is applied, it is by central governmental authorities. In the larger cities and some towns, the government operates public general hospitals staffed by salaried doctors and other personnel. Also, health centers for ambulatory care, both therapeutic and preventive, have been established in the cities and at some trade centers of rural regions. These facilities and often smaller peripheral health stations are staffed mainly by auxiliary health personnel with very limited training, and only occasionally by doctors. When physicians are available outside the cities, they are typically expected to supervise the health care of huge populations of 50,000 to 100,000.

Since there are only very small proportions of industrial workers with regular wages, there are neither social insurance nor voluntary insurance programs for medical care. Here and there, a large corporation in mining or agricultural production may operate a closed system of health services for its workers and their families. Also, in a handful of rural locations, there may be religious missions offering semicharitable medical care for small payments by the people. Dr. Albert Schweitzer's improvised hospital at Lambarene, in former French Equatorial Africa (now Gabon), was a famous example of this pattern, now dying out.

Since many underdeveloped countries are tropical, the people suffer from rampant vector-borne diseases such as malaria or filariasis, and even the nontropical countries have very high rates of tuberculosis, leprosy, and other chronic infectious diseases. To tackle these scourges, central governments typically mount disease control or eradication campaigns, but these are seldom built on any infrastructure of local health services. Demonstrations of model health programs, usually with foreign assistance, are seen here and there, such as at Danfa near the capital city (Accra) of Ghana. Most of these special projects are close to an urban center, where a medical school may use the demonstration unit for training purposes.

In the main cities, there is typically a heavy concentration of the limited supply of physicians and dentists in the country. These practitioners serve the handful of wealthy families and usually work part of their time in the urban hospitals, where they also serve the low-income city dwellers for severe disorders. There are usually numerous pharmacies, often operated by traditional healers such as Chinese herbalists, where poor people go directly for medications to cope with their symptoms.

The number of doctors and the supply of health facilities in the underdeveloped countries have been slowly improving. These, often with the aid of international agencies, are engaged in planning the output of more health care resources and are applying various strategies to get health services to the rural populations. With the tradition of previous colonial authority systems, the national plans usually call for highly organized networks of health facilities, making great use of briefly trained auxiliary personnel. The tasks that lie ahead are always tremendous.

Transitional Systems

Many still predominantly agricultural and rural countries have made much progress in developing their health care systems, which may properly be defined as transitional. The approximately twenty republics of Latin America belong generally in this category, as do certain countries of the Middle East, such as Iran, Turkey, or Lebanon.

In these countries, although the majority of the population still live under very poor conditions, a modest structure of organized health services has usually been developed. In Latin America the influential Catholic church established numerous charitable hospitals many years ago. Ministries of health have built additional modern hospitals, as well as quite extensive networks of health centers and health stations in both urban and rural districts. In the most isolated rural areas, traditional healers and midwives still tend patients, but they are being noticeably replaced by scientific resources. Pharmacies remain the source of much self-medication, but they sell imported pharmaceuticals more than herbal remedies.

Most important, all these countries have made beginnings in social insurance systems to support medical care for industrial workers and often their dependents. Although these are typically only a small fraction of national populations—around 10 to 15 percent—their proportions are rising. Rather well-staffed and equipped hospitals and health centers (or polyclinics with specialists) are established for insured beneficiaries. Unlike the pattern of social insurance in the European welfare states, doctors and others provide both the ambulatory and inpatient care on salaries and under organized arrangements. Various types of coordination are being developed between these social security programs and those of health ministries and welfare societies.

For the affluent a substantial private medical sector still functions. Most of the doctors, who serve on salaries in the organized health programs, are also engaged in private practice for part of each day. Training institutions are turning out doctors and other health personnel at accelerating rates, so that the ratio of physicians to population is improving. One finds a doctor for each 2,000 to 6,000 Latin American people (in Argentina, more than one doctor per 800), in contrast to ratios of one doctor to 20,000 or 60,000 people in the underdeveloped systems. Yet, the distribution of doctors typically remains uneven, with the concentration being in the largest cities.

Changes are occurring rapidly in the health care systems of these transitional countries. Many doctors and others go to North America or Europe for further specialized training, not only in clinical medicine but also in public health work. In Latin America there are ten schools of public health to train manpower for administration of the organized health care systems. Favored groups, such as military personnel or governmental officials, are often served by special highly developed subsystems of preventive and curative medicine.

Socialist Systems

Since the Russian Revolution of 1917 there has arisen in the world a markedly different type of health care system. Embodying the political principles of socialism, health care has become essentially a public service, with almost all personnel employed as civil servants and all facilities owned and operated by the government. Health service theoretically is a right of citizenship.

The concepts of socialism applied to health care were developed over the first twenty years or so after the Russian Revolution. A high priority was assigned to health, especially for workers and for children, and remarkably large numbers of doctors and others were rapidly trained. Hospitals, polyclinics, and health centers were built, and the new graduates were employed in them on state salaries. As the public system was developed, private medical and dental practice gradually declined, although it has not disappeared entirely. Organizationally, no distinction was made in the responsibilities for prevention and for treatment; each doctor and each health facility was expected to do both.

The problem of rural health manpower, so common throughout the world, was tackled in various ways. Since all medical students were trained at public expense, including coverage of their living costs while at school, every graduate was required to spend three years at a rural post. If he or she (a majority of doctors are women) volunteered to remain after this, a higher salary would be earned than at an urban post. As the numbers of doctors and other personnel increased and as an administrative structure for health service was built up everywhere, finding employment would depend on a person's going where there were openings. If the city positions were filled, health personnel would naturally go to a rural area without being ordered to do so. This strategy has not equalized the urban-rural doctor distribution in the Soviet Union completely, but with a large supply of such auxiliary personnel as nurses, midwives, and *feldshers* (field assistants), it has achieved greater equity than in other large countries.

After the first turbulent years, Soviet health services, like most other aspects of Soviet life, became subject to systematic planning. For each five-year period, certain goals were set with respect to the production of resources and their distribution. Norms were established by a central planning agency to define the ratios of personnel and other resources needed; for example, the optimal standard for doctors in the USSR has been about 1 to 330 people, and with a current ratio of 1 to 400 (a much higher ratio than in the United States) it is nearly achieved. Hospitals were likewise planned according to a regionalized scheme of central, intermediate, and peripheral facilities, with graded technical responsibilities.

Since virtually all health service responsibility was in the hands of government, it was assigned to a unified Ministry of Health rather than to different authorities. A hierarchy of branches of this ministry operate at the peripheral levels—republic, province (*oblast*), and district (*rayon*). Under the Soviet Health Ministry is responsibility not only for all health services, preventive and therapeutic, but also for health-related functions that, in all the other types of health systems, come under other sponsorships. This includes the education of all health personnel, which in 1937 was transferred from the Ministry of Education. It includes the manufacture (or decisions on manufacture) of all drugs, supplies, and medical equipment. It includes also the conduct of all research through the Academy of Medical Sciences and hundreds of component branch institutes.

This socialist model of health services, pioneered in the Soviet Union, has been emulated with various modificatic.ıs in the "people's democracies" of eastern Europe. Each of these other socialist countries naturally has had to make certain adjustments to its local circumstances. In Poland, for example, an appreciable private sector operated in the rural areas for a long time. In Czechoslovakia, the university medical schools were not transferred to the health ministry. When a socialist revolution took place in Cuba in 1959, the basic Soviet model was gradually adopted, but with Cuba being such a small country, less authority was delegated peripherally than in the huge USSR.

When China had its revolution (or "liberation," as the Chinese people call it) in 1949, it also initially adopted the Soviet system. After the political break with the USSR in 1960, however, and especially after the Proletarian Cultural Revolution of 1966-1970, the pattern was changed considerably. For so tremendous a population (700,000,000 to 800,000,000 people), the relatively bureaucratic and hierarchical Soviet pattern did not prove to be so effective. Severe deficiencies remained in the rural areas nearly twenty years after the revolution. Therefore, decentralized initiative (still under the guidance of the Communist Party) was emphasized, with the slogan of "local self-reliance." Great stress was put on a minimal but widely available level of health care for the rural population through the rapid training of thousands of peasants as "barefoot doctors." These health workers treat minor ailments and promote prevention (including family planning) at the level of each rural "production brigade," which consists of from 500 to 3,000 people.

Thus, the socialist type of health care system, like each of the other systems we have discussed, takes somewhat different forms in each country. Its common feature is the establishment of health care as a responsibility of some level of government (including the Chinese rural commune) and a right of every resident, even though for certain services the individual may normally have to make small personal payments. (In the USSR, for example, some payments are still expected for drugs and certain types of dental care; in China, small fees are commonly required for ambulatory services in rural areas; in Yugoslavia, there is still an appreciable sector of private medical practice.) The goal in all socialist systems, however, is to make complete health services available to everyone without charge.

Each of the five principal types of health care system is distinguishable from the others, even though each also has variations within its own type. Over time, changes are occurring in all the systems. If we think of the countries within each category as illustrating a continuum of patterns, we can understand that at the extremes a national system may eventually develop into another category. Australia, for example, has recently been moving from the free enterprise to the welfare state pattern; Egypt may be moving from the underdeveloped to the transitional pattern; Costa Rica seems to be evolving from the transitional to the welfare state pattern; Great Britain is in many ways moving from the welfare state to the socialist pattern (even in the absence of a social revolution).

Although these judgments may be debatable, this rough classification of the types of health care system in the different nations of the world should simplify the examination of the various aspects of a system in the chapters that follow. Instead of examining the total efforts to provide and improve health care on a country-by-country basis, we will take an overview of these definable features of a system as they are illustrated in countries of each type throughout the world. What are the main features by which a health care system may be analyzed?

The Components of a Health Care System

There are doubtless many ways of describing a health care system. We will use a scheme of analysis with seven principal components.

1. Economic Support Since the methods by which health services are financed are basic determinants of their quantity, their quality, and their impact on people, we will consider these first. Six fundamental mechanisms of individual and collective financing are definable and, although all of them are used to some extent in almost every country, their proportions differ greatly.

2. Manpower Historically the healing of the sick was the province of one type of person, the doctor, but as medicine has developed, a great number and variety of more specialized health workers have evolved. Their functions, training, and the social controls of their performance must be considered as these features have taken shape in different nations.

3. Facilities To shelter and care for the seriously sick, hospitals have developed in all countries. Their sponsorships, mode of operation, relative numbers, and relationships to other components of health service differ greatly in various national settings. Other types of structure, such as health centers for service to the ambulatory person, have also multiplied and these may be reviewed around the world.

4. Delivery Patterns Perhaps the most striking differences among nations are in the patterns by which health services are provided or delivered. The same

types of manpower and facilities or even the same mechanisms of financial support may be applied, but the methods by which the work is carried out show
great variation. These patterns of delivery of medical care, which include the
ways that personnel and facilities are paid, have large implications for the cost
and quality of services.

   5. Preventive Services It was centuries before medical science matured
in its understanding of disease processes and health sufficiently to learn how to
prevent sickness. The techniques for prevention depend, of course, on the nature
of the disease problems in different countries and the characteristics of the health
care system. These are components of health service with generally rising
importance.

   6. Regulation Every complex system of manpower and facilities requires
some regulation or surveillance to keep it effective and to assure the attainment
of its goals with the greatest possible efficiency. The many ways that this is done
in different national contexts have diverse influences in the functioning of the
health care system.

   7. Administration and Planning Finally, to manage whole systems of
health service, to keep them supplied with economic support and resources, and
to assure their effective operation requires some sort of over-all supervision.
Planning for the future also requires deliberate efforts. These methods of administration depend on the prevailing political and economic structures of various
nations.

   Beyond these seven basic components in every health care system, the
course of developments in all countries has been influenced to varying extents
by actions across national borders. Some international actions are private,
others are governmental. Some involve interchanges between two countries or
perhaps a few; others constitute the work of world-wide international agencies.
A review of these cross-national health activities is clearly relevant. Finally, to
get some idea of what probably lies ahead in the world, it can be helpful to
take a bird's-eye view of broad past trends. If we can detect any general tendencies in numerous countries, we may be able to predict the likely course of
future events in any particular country. Such an overview may serve also to
summarize the highlights of major past and current efforts to provide health
care in the nations of the world.

Readings

Abel-Smith, Brian, *An International Study of Health Expenditures, and Its Relevance for Health Planning,* Geneva: World Health Organization, Public Health Papers No. 32, 1967

Blum, Richard and Eva Blum, *Health and Healing in Rural Greece,* Stanford: Stanford University Press, 1965.

Bryant, John, *Health and the Developing World,* Ithaca, N.Y.: Cornell University Press, 1969.

Crozier, Ralph C., "Medicine, Modernization and Cultural Crisis in China and India," *Comparative Studies and History, 12*: 275-291 (July 1970).

Dubos, René, *Man Adapting,* New Haven: Yale University Press, 1965.

Eckstein, Harry, *The English Health Service: Its Origins, Structures, and Achievements,* Cambridge, Mass.: Harvard University Press.

Elling, Ray H., "Case Studies of Contrasting Approaches to Organizing for Health: An Introduction to a Framework," *Social Science and Medicine, 8*: 263-270 (1974).

Evang, Karl, *Health Service, Society, and Medicine,* London: Oxford University Press, 1960.

Fanon, Frantz, "Colonialism and Health," in *The Wretched of the Earth,* New York: Grove Press, 1965.

Foster, G. M., *Problems of Intercultural Health Programs,* New York: Social Science Research Council, 1958.

Fry, John and W. A. J. Farndale (eds.), *International Medical Care: A Comparison and Evaluation of Medical Care Services Throughout the World:* Oxford: Medical and Technical Publishing Co., 1972.

Gabaldon, A., "Health Services and Socio-Economic Development in Latin America," *The Lancet, 4* December 1969, pp. 739-746.

Kohn, R. and S. Radius, "International Comparisons of Health Service Systems— An Annotated Bibliography," *International Journal of Health Services, 3:* 295-309 (1973).

Liang, Matthiew et al., "Chinese Health Care: Determinants of the System," *American Journal of Public Health, 63*: 102-110 (February 1973).

Litman, T. J. and L. Robins, "Comparative Analysis of Health Care Systems— A Socio-political Approach," *Social Science and Medicine, 5*: 573-581 (1971).

Malenbaum, W., "Health and Economic Expansion in Poor Lands," *International Journal of Health Services, 3*: 161-176 (1973).

Marmor, Theodore R., *The Politics of Medicare,* Chicago: Aldine Publishing Co., 1973.

McNamara, Robert, *One Hundred Countries, Two Billion People: The Dimensions of Development,* New York: Praeger Publishers, 1973.

Mechanic, David, *Politics, Medicine, and Social Science,* New York: John Wiley and Sons, 1974.

Myrdal, Gunnar, *The Challenge of World Poverty*, New York: Vintage Books, 1970.

National Council for International Health, *Selected Sources of Information in International Health Areas*, Chicago: NICH, 1973.

Navarro, Vicente, "What Does Chile Mean: An Analysis of Events in the Health Sector Before, During, and After Allende's Administration," *Health and Society, 52*:93-130 (Spring 1974).

——, "Social Policy Issues: An Explanation of the Composition, Nature, and Functions of the Present Health Sector of the United States," *Bulletin of the New York Academy of Medicine, 51*:199-234 (January 1975).

——, "The Underdevelopment of Health or the Health of Underdevelopment: An Analysis of the Distribution of Human Health Resources in Latin America," *International Journal of Health Services, 4*:5-27 (1974).

Onoge, O. F., "Capitalism and Public Health: A Neglected Theme in the Medical Anthropology of Africa," in *Topias and Utopias in Health: Policy Studies*, S. R. Ingnam and A. E. Thomas (eds.), The Hague: Mouton Publishers, 1975.

Roemer, Milton I., "Political Ideology and Health Care: Hospital Patterns in the Philippines and Cuba," *International Journal of Health Services, 3*:487-492 (1973).

Sand, René, *The Advance to Social Medicine*, London: Staples Press, 1952.

Sax, Sidney, *Medical Care in the Melting Pot—An Australian Review*, Melbourne: Angus and Robertson, 1972.

Seham, Max, "An American Doctor Looks at Eleven Foreign Health Systems," *Social Science and Medicine, 3*:65-81 (1969).

Shenkin, Budd N., "Politics and Medical Care in Sweden: The Seven Crowns Reform," *New England Journal of Medicine, 288*:555-559 (March 1973).

Sigerist, Henry E., *Civilization and Disease*, Ithaca, N.Y.: Cornell University Press, 1943.

——, "War and Medicine," *Journal of Laboratory and Clinical Medicine, 28*: 531-538 (February 1943).

——, "Nationalism and Internationalism in Medicine," *Bulletin of the History of Medicine, 21*:5-16 (January-February 1947).

——, *On the Sociology of Medicine*, M. I. Roemer (ed.), New York: MD Publications, 1960.

Silver, George A., *A Spy in the House of Medicine*, Germantown, Md.: Aspen Systems Corp., 1976.

Weinerman, E. Richard, "Research on Comparative Health Service Systems," *Medical Care, 9*:272-290 (May-June 1971).

White, Kerr L., "International Comparisons of Health Service Systems," *Milbank Memorial Fund Quarterly, 46*:117-125, Part 2 (April 1968).

2

ECONOMIC SUPPORT FOR HEALTH SERVICES

In all societies there is an economic aspect to health services. The personnel, facilities, and supplies used for the treatment or prevention of disease must be financed in some way. The methods of financing, however, are highly variable among countries and also within countries. They vary with the general structure of the economic system and the degree to which it follows free market rules as against systematic planning. They also vary with political ideologies and the attitudes toward certain diseases or population groups.

This chapter will help you to understand the diversity of methods by which health services are financed in different economic and political settings. It will also clarify the implications of these methods for the quantity and quality of health services provided. Economic support is not simply a matter of money and accounting; it is a basic determinant of the whole character of the health service system as well.

Introduction

There are hundreds of ways by which health services have been financed at different times and places. Broadly speaking they can be classified into six types:

1. Personal payment Personal payment is the private purchase of services through the individual's personal resources, including money he may have borrowed or received from another source (a relative, friend, loan company, or the like). Personal payment can also include payment by barter.

2. Charity Charity consists of support from funds or work donated voluntarily by persons who are different from the beneficiaries of the service.

3. *Payment by Industry*   Payment by industry is the provision of services out of the earnings of an enterprise, typically for the workers in that
establishment.

4. *Voluntary insurance*   Voluntary insurance supports medical services
with funds raised through periodic personal contributions of groups of people
before sickness strikes. There may be various sorts of nongovernmental sponsorship, but the services are financed only for the contributors and sometimes their
dependents.

5. *Social insurance*   Social insurance consists of periodic contributions
required by law to support certain services to designated beneficiaries. Statutory
requirements may establish earmarked governmental funds or may mandate
insurance contributions to various nonofficial bodies.

6. *General revenues*   General revenues support health services through
various forms of taxation on land, incomes, sales, corporation profits, imports,
or the like. These taxes may be levied by different levels of government—national, provincial, local, or other—and the services ordinarily bear no relation to the
taxpayers.
It is evident that under each of these main methods of financing there are
many variations. It may be noted that the different methods follow a sort of
spectrum moving from very individualistic to increasingly cooperative or collective approaches. In the majority of countries, all six methods will be utilized in
providing health services for certain sectors of the population or for dealing
with certain diseases, but the proportionate mix varies greatly. In general, the
methods at the individualistic end of the range are more important in countries
dominated by free market economies, such as the United States, whereas methods
at the collectivist end are more important in centrally planned economies, such as
the Soviet Union. Between these two extremes are a great many countries with
very mixed or transitional economic systems and corresponding patterns of economic support for health services.

Personal Payment

Personal payment for health services is found to some degree in all countries,
even in those with highly socialized economies. Hardly anywhere, however, is
this the predominant method. Even in the United States, with its free market
economy, private support for medical services ceased being the predominant
financing method about fifteen to twenty years ago; since then, a combination
of various group-financing methods has come to predominate.

The private payment method means that health service is distributed, as are other commodities, on the basis of individual purchasing power rather than on needs stemming from the illness itself. Thus, individuals of higher income generally obtain more services, although for many reasons they tend to have less illness. It is this very inequity, of course, that has led increasingly to the replacement of this method by the several more collectivized methods.

Countries with highly developed systems of social insurance or social security for supporting health service (Sweden, for example) still leave room for a private support sector. Some few people may choose to see a private specialist outside the system and pay him personally at a rate higher than the official rate. In addition, the official system in Sweden and many other countries with social insurance (to be discussed later) requires that the patient assumè part of the cost. A fixed amount or a percentage (commonly 20 percent) of the official charge is payable by the patient rather than by the insurance fund.

Even in the socialist countries such as the Soviet Union, a small private sector remains. A very small fraction of people—perhaps 1 or 2 percent—who have the money and do not wish to wait their turn in a clinic or hospital will pay a doctor personally for special attention that is typically given after the doctor's official working hours. Naturally, the more fully a public system meets the health needs of people, the less are they likely to resort to privately financed care.

However, these fractional portions of privately financed health service in predominantly socially supported health care systems are unimportant compared with private payment in countries where the public system is quite weak. Private payment predominates for certain services, like ambulatory care by physicians and dentists or for medications, in the United States. Although hospitalization and inpatient medical and surgical services are now predominantly financed by voluntary or social insurance programs, ordinary office and home care, dental services, and drugs are insured benefits for only a small percentage of the American population. Hence, the cost of these services make up most of the approximately 40 percent of health care costs in the United States still borne by purely private payments.

In the less developed countries in Africa, Latin America, and Asia, the private sector constitutes a still greater share of the medical market, even though it usually involves only a small minority of the people. In countries such as Ethiopia, Ecuador, or Thailand—to choose one from each of these three continents—there may be only 10 percent or less of the population who can pay for modern medical services privately. This affluent minority get the lion's share of the nation's health service resources for their personal benefit. The great majority of the population must depend on socially financed services that absorb a lesser portion of the total medical resources. These inequitable relationships may be represented by Fig. 1.

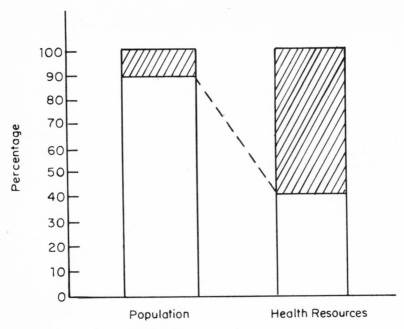

FIGURE 1   Distribution of health resources in a developing country.

In other words, a relatively wealthy 10 percent of the population in these impoverished nations spend the money to purchase 60 percent of the services of doctors, hospitals, nurses, and so on. This affluent minority of people are usually concentrated in a few large cities. Meanwhile, through taxation (usually modest in rates and inadequately collected) and other social devices, 40 percent of the available health care resources are devoted to organized programs on which 90 percent of the population must depend. This schema is an oversimplification, and the proportions are indeed changing as the social and political consciousness of people rises. However, it represents the relationships now prevailing in many developing countries.

The schema, as noted, refers to "modern medical services," that is, the services of scientifically trained personnel and rationally designed facilities or scientifically prepared equipment and supplies. To some extent the imbalance is adjusted by numerous small expenditures of poor village dwellers on traditional healers. Payment by barter or by very low fees is made to indigenous "doctors" or midwives in rural areas of the less developed countries from the private re-sources of families, and these outlays must be counted also as part of the private sector. The therapeutic value of this primitive medicine is still the subject of scientific research. Some of the village practices, derived from empirical observations over the centuries, may be effective, especially with respect to psychosomatic disorders.

It is contended by some that personal payment or some financial sacrifice by the patient contributes to the effectiveness of medical care. What the patient does not directly pay for, it is argued, he does not appreciate, and it will not work as well. All economic support of health services is ultimately from the people, and as social mechanisms for financing health care expand, this contention is heard less often. In Great Britain, for example, where the vast bulk of health service is socially financed, there is no evidence that it is less well appreciated by patients. In fact, all the opinion surveys show that the British have a higher degree of satisfaction with their health services than Americans do with theirs.

Charity

From the early Christian era, charitable donations, often inspired by religious motives, have supported health services for the poor. The construction of the first hospitals in Europe, as well as their initial operating costs, were supported by bequests from the wealthy. Such generosity tended not only to prove the piety of the donor, helping to pave a pathway for him to an afterlife in heaven, but also strengthened his voice in the affairs of the church or the hospital here on earth.

As medical science advanced and as the staffing and equipment of hospitals deemed necessary for the proper care of patients increased, the costs of hospital operations gradually rose. To keep going, hospitals had to turn to other sources for additional financial support—first to local governments, then to payments from patients, much later to social insurance. Meantime, as feudalism declined and a middle class of merchants and artisans arose, modest charitable donations were derived from greater numbers of people. With the advance of the industrial revolution and the Enlightment, charity became the financial source for supporting other health services, such as the care of crippled children or the purchase of food for the poor.

In the nineteenth century, with the sharper identification of numerous disease entities, voluntary societies were organized by well-to-do people for tackling tuberculosis or for reducing infant mortality or for furnishing the services of visiting nurses to the homes of the poor. Scores of such societies were financed first by charity, although later they derived funds from government and other sources. The Red Cross, inspired obviously by the cross of Christ, was organized to give help in all sorts of emergencies, in time of war, or in catastrophes due to "acts of God." One finds today in all countries—although more in the industrialized and affluent nations—hundreds of voluntary agencies organized for dealing with particular diseases or for furnishing certain types of service. As personal health services have come to be financed in other ways, these charity-supported bodies have often shifted their objectives to the promotion of medical research or training.

In the less developed countries, it is common for a private health care organization to be launched by prestigious social figures such as the wife of the president or the king. This organization soon attracts the voluntary services of other upper-class women and sometimes men. A small program may be launched for providing milk to malnourished children or for operating ambulances or for giving prenatal care to mothers of low income. Then, to expand the services, government is called upon to subsidize them. In time, the great bulk of support is derived from public sources, although management of the clinics, the hospitals, the vehicles, and so on remains with private boards of directors. In nearly all less developed countries, the Red Cross societies, although nongovernmental, are financed today mainly by public revenue sources.

In both the industrialized and the developing worlds, hospitals are still often controlled by boards of citizens chosen by successive generations of voluntary, charitable donors. The hospitals often retain their saintly or other sacred names long after the costs of their operation, and even sometimes their effective authorities, have been transferred to government hands. In Latin America, where the Catholic church has been a powerful force, the hospitals of *beneficencia* or welfare societies of charitable origins are still autonomous even when their financial support and standards of operation have become responsibilities of government.

As a percentage of the total monies used for the support of health services, charitable donations have generally declined. In the United States, where national economic data are more available than in most other countries, the proportion is down to 2 or 3 percent. Yet this small fraction can be important in the launching or testing of new ideas for health service, scientific education, or research. The concept of special sanatoria for treating tuberculosis, first tested in nineteenth century Germany through charitable financing, is an illustration. The development of the first poliomyelitis vaccine by Salk was financed by the charitable March of Dimes program in America. Infant health stations were pioneered by French charities. As the value of such innovations is proven, stronger and more stable financial support is attracted from government and other sources.

The sliding scale of medical fees referred to earlier has been, in a sense, another form of charity by individual doctors who serve low-income patients for reduced fees or even without charge, while they collect much higher fees from the wealthy. This practice was much more common in previous decades before government programs were developed to pay doctors and others for services to the poor. It is still customary, however, for hospitals to expect private doctors to serve outpatients and also some indigent inpatients without remuneration, in exchange for the privilege of having accessibility to hospital beds for their private paying patients from whom they receive lucrative fees.

Religious missions, either domestic or foreign, are another form of charity often providing health services. Missions from Western Europe or North America to Africa, Latin America, or Asia have established hundreds of hospitals and health stations staffed with trained doctors and nurses. Although their primary objective is religious conversion, they provide health services as a means to this end. Usually they make small charges to the local people for services, and they may also become subsidized by national governments. As former colonies have become emancipated, the mission personnel are often sent away by the new governments, but their physical facilities may be integrated into the public system.

Philanthropic foundations are another form of charity support for health services both at home and abroad. Bodies like the Rockefeller or Ford Foundations in the United States, the Nuffield Trust in England, or the Rothschild endowments in France have supported hundreds of health projects all over the world. Innovations as diverse as the first comprehensive health center in rural Sri Lanka, formerly Ceylon (Kalutara in 1924), the integrated pattern of medical education at Western Reserve University (Cleveland, Ohio), a training program for hospital administrators (London, England), or a demonstration community health program (near Jerusalem, Israel) have been launched with foundation grants. The declining proportionate role of charity in health service financing is owed not to any absolute reduction in the amount of voluntary donations for health purposes but rather to the greatly increased monies derived from other sources.

Finally in recent years, village people in less developed and socialist countries have contributed voluntary labor to building rural health centers and promoting health campaigns.

Industry

Maintenance of high economic productivity requires a healthy population of workers, so that large enterprises have long found it efficient to provide certain health services to their employees. In advanced industrial nations, most health care needs of workers and others are met by resources in the general community, so that industrial enterprises ordinarily finance only the care of on-the-job injuries or illnesses. In the less developed countries, general community resources are seldom adequate, so that a large corporation may finance and provide over-all health care for its workers and often for their families as well.

Even in the wealthy United States, industries isolated from urban life, such as certain mines, lumber companies, and the railroads in their period of initial construction, often have found it necessary to organize and finance general medical care for their workers because no local doctors or hospitals were available. Sometimes the money for this service has been derived from wage-deductions (a form of non-governmental insurance), but sometimes it has been solely or partly contributed by management.

In the less developed countries, management support of general health services for workers, at least in large enterprises, has been more common. The exploitation of natural resources for foreign export, usually by foreign-owned companies, was so profitable and local wages typically so low, that corporate assumption of these costs was relatively inexpensive. The oil companies in Saudi Arabia, the rubber plantations in Liberia, the banana *fincas* in Guatemala, the copper mines in Chile, and the large tea estates in Ceylon typically finance general medical care programs for their employees. In many such countries, laws have been enacted requiring health services to be provided by firms employing over 100 workers.

Since 1885, when Germany passed the first industrial injury insurance act, such measures have been legislated by most countries with any degree of industrial development. These laws, first enacted in the United States in 1910 on a state-by-state basis, are called workmen's compensation laws. In general, they require employers to take financial responsibility for the cost of injuries that occur on the job and occupational diseases, by compensating the worker both for loss of wages from the resultant disability and by paying the costs of needed medical care. Employers typically buy insurance, through either private insurance companies or a government insurance fund, to meet such contingencies. Ordinarily, the premiums payable by employers depend on the accident rate and the severity of the disabilities caused, a policy called experience rating.

As a result of the policy of experience rating, the industrial injury insurance acts have offered a financial inducement to employers to design their workplaces in consideration of the worker's safety. Also, to minimize complications after an injury occurs, companies are encouraged to provide emergency medical services at or near the workplace. By pre-employment and thereafter periodic medical examinations of workers, it can be determined whether a worker is physically fit for various types of jobs. Numerous problems surround the services of industrial physicians. Possibly involved may be the personal welfare of the worker which may be contrary to the financial interests of the employer. However, the relevant point here is that the financing of these services is assumed by management as part of the costs of production.

In the socialist countries, first in the Soviet Union and later in others, health services at the workplace have been customarily provided on a broad scale. That is, little or no distinction is made between the treatment of job-related disorders and any others. Since government owns and operates the industries and likewise finances general health services in the community, there is no reason to avoid competition with private medical practice—a philosophy that dominates policies in most capitalist countries. Large factories and other work-places in the socialist countries often maintain health care systems for the workers as a feature of the production environment.

In France following World War II, the first law was passed outside the socialist countries mandating all employers to engage physicians and nurses to serve workers. There are legally defined standards—for example, one full-time doctor for 500 workers and proportionate part-time doctors for smaller numbers. To meet the legal requirements, several small plants often combine to finance the services of one or more doctors and nurses. Belgium and a few other countries have since passed similar legislation.

As a share of over-all national costs of health services, the financial responsibilities assumed by industry are not very great—usually less than 5 percent of the total. Nevertheless, they constitute a form of social financing through which the economic burden is spread widely among all the parties that purchase the products of a company because the health services simply become part of the costs of production. Closely related, but distinguishable in their economic impact, are the contributions of management to the costs of general health insurance for workers—either voluntarily or by law. This type of financing is considered in the next section.

Voluntary Insurance

In the late Middle Ages, guilds of artisans were formed—masons, barbers, silver-smiths, and so on—to establish standards of skill and protect the financial interests of the trade. Among other things, the guilds also provided for the personal welfare of their members by pooling funds to meet various adversities such as old age or sickness. Personal welfare protection meant replacement of earnings lost owing to disability and payment of the costs of medical care. This early type of voluntary health insurance took another form in the eighteenth and nineteenth centuries when industries developed that employed many workers. Instead of having the independence of a free artisan or tradesman, the worker became totally dependent on wages for his survival. To protect himself and his family from the risk of sickness he joined with other workers in cooperatives that could replace part of the wages lost during sickness and meet the costs of drugs and a doctor's care. Hospitalization was sought only as a last resort, and this was provided free in public or charitable facilities. Sometimes employers encouraged their workers to join these "sickness chests" (*Krankenkassen* in Germany) by also contributing money to them. These chests helped to maintain healthy and productive workers, and they also lightened the load on charity or public revenues if the worker became sick to the point of indigency.

Throughout the nineteenth century, sickness insurance or mutual benefit societies grew rapidly throughout Europe. In Great Britain they were called friendly societies, in France *mutualités*. Sometimes they were organized simply on a geographic basis, being open to working people of any type in one community. Sometimes there were societies covering a particular occupation, such as coal miners or textile workers, in a large region. In some countries, the societies defined membership eligibility along religious or political lines. Laws were sometimes passed prescribing rules to protect the financial solvency of the funds and hence the rights of their members. Some sickness societies engaged one or more doctors to provide care to the members for fixed monthly payments, perhaps calculated on a per capita basis. Others paid any doctor consulted on a fee basis.

The concept of mutual benefit societies was transmitted to the United States in the late nineteenth and early twentieth centuries by immigrants from Europe. Mutual benefit societies were formed in many large cities, especially New York and Boston. Often the groupings were on the basis of the person's country of origin and were designated as fraternal orders. In the highly mobile and changing American economy, however, these voluntary health insurance organizations never achieved the stability or importance found in Europe. Many of them failed when the financial claims on them exceeded the funds that had been periodically contributed.

A different pattern emerged in the United States when commercial insurance companies began to sell group insurance for life or funeral benefits to all the workers in any particular firm. In the early twentieth century the insurance companies extended the concept to partial replacement of wages in cases of accident or serious illness. These health and accident insurance policies were sometimes partially financed by employers as a paternalistic fringe benefit, often to discourage unionization. It was very rare, however, for commercial carriers to cover the cost of hospital or medical care for the disability for which they insured part of wage losses.

A turning point occurred in 1929 when an organization of teachers in Dallas, Texas, pooled small periodic contributions to build a fund that would pay the cost of hospitalization for any member needing it. This was the year of onset of the Great Depression; hospitals all over the country soon found their beds half empty and their accounts in the red. The Dallas idea, therefore, seemed very attractive to the hospitals as well as the population in many places. Similar hospitalization plans were organized in New Jersey, Michigan, and elsewhere. By 1934, the American Hospital Association backed up the idea, offered a set of standards for such insurance plans, and gave the movement a symbol— the Blue Cross. Thousands, then millions, of working people became enrolled as groups in Blue Cross plans that paid all or most of the cost of hospitalization.

At first the American medical profession viewed this movement with alarm and opposed it as an entering wedge of socialized medicine. After a few years, however, doctors recognized its value and, in fact, decided to emulate the idea with insurance organizations sponsored by medical societies to pay surgical (later medical) fees in hospitalized cases. Starting in California in 1939 this movement soon gained momentum and spread elsewhere under the symbol of a Blue Shield. These programs, like the Blue Cross plans, were usually organized on a state-by-state basis and eventually they cooperated with one another in marketing, claims processing, and so on. Sometimes a Blue Shield plan paid for certain out-of-hospital doctor services, but this was exceptional.

With the success of the Blue Cross and Blue Shield movements, the commercial insurance companies changed their viewpoint. They also began to sell group insurance to pay for hospital and medical costs as well as for wage replacement. Their marketing methods were so effective—especially in their sale of "packages" of insurance for life, disability, old-age pensions, and so on, as well as medical care costs—that by the 1960s they had overtaken the Blue Cross and Blue Shield plans in their total enrollment. Instead of paying hospital and doctor bills directly, the commercial companies indemnified the insured person with a certain sum, which might or might not be enough to pay the bill. Thus, the patient was often left with a sizeable financial load, despite his insurance, but this strategy provided the companies with a hedge against rising medical costs. Through the indemnification principle, the insurance companies could keep their premiums stable, whereas the "Blue" plans, paying full service benefits, had to raise their premiums and lost out in the competition for health insurance buyers.

This American pattern of insurance, sponsored by the providers of health care and by private insurance companies instead of consumers, has been almost unique in the world scene. In the 1950s it was emulated in Australia and to a minor extent in other industrialized countries. Voluntary insurance in Europe, where it began, was sponsored predominantly by groups of workers or other consumers.

The European sickness insurance societies grew steadily in scope, both in the numbers and types of persons they covered and in the range of medical services for which they provided financial protection. In 1883 a major turning point occurred, when Germany passed the first law *requiring* that workers below a certain income level must become enrolled in a sickness insurance society. This was the birth of social insurance, to be discussed later, but apropos of voluntary insurance another fact should be noted here. This is that, even after enrollment in an insurance fund became compulsory for certain persons (typically workers of low income), other people could still enroll in these programs voluntarily. This was done by thousands of higher income families. Today in many countries where social insurance legislation encompasses the majority of a national population (perhaps 80 or 90 percent), many of the remaining 10 or 20 percent of people are voluntarily insured through the same organizations.

Voluntary health insurance has many implications for medical care besides the lightening of financial burdens at times of sickness. Perhaps most important is the easier accessibility to care, when an illness is not far advanced, with costs spread in this way. At the same time, the collective and socially visible financing invariably leads to greater constraints or controls on the provision of services than those that prevail in the open medical market. This influences both quality and costs. Because of heightened demands, there are impacts also on the supply and distribution of health manpower, facilities, and supplies. These and other ramifications of insurance financing are more fully discussed elsewhere, but now we must consider the next form of economic support for health care—social insurance.

Social Insurance

The 1883 law of Germany mentioned earlier ushered in a movement for mandatory insurance against several social risks. This movement has now become world-wide. In the United States, since the crucial legislation of 1935, it has become known as Social Security. The Social Security Act applied originally to the provision of pensions in old age, to insurance for survivors of a deceased worker (life insurance), and to compensation during periods of unemployment. In the 1950s insurance protection against total long-term disability was added, and in 1965 the principal costs of hospital and medical care for pensioners—the Medicare program—were brought under the U.S. Social Security umbrella.

Other countries, mainly in Europe but also in Latin America, the Middle East, and elsewhere, followed the pioneering example of Germany for insurance of medical costs in earlier periods. Soon after Germany's action, Austria and Hungary followed suit, then the Scandinavian countries, Great Britain in 1911, and eventually every European country. Each of the national programs differed in the types and proportion of population covered, the exact scope of health services financed, the methods of administration, and so on. All the European systems of social insurance for medical care were similar, however, in being built on the earlier framework of voluntary health insurance bodies. The laws basically required that workers with incomes below a stated level (often excluding such categories as agricultural workers or domestic servants) must be insured for designated medical care costs through an approved organization. The approval of the various insurance societies was a central government responsibility, usually through a ministry of labor or of welfare. To be approved, the society had to meet certain standards of administration, of services or benefits financed, of costs, of enrollment policies, and so on.

In some countries and in the earlier laws, each insurance society collected the periodic premiums and paid out the charges for medical care. In other countries and in the later laws, the collection of insurance contributions was done by the central government which, in turn, allocated money out to the different societies in accordance with their enrollments. The payment of medical and related bills was then made by the local society. In all countries, insurance contributions were required from the employers as well as the workers, and sometimes there was a contribution from government as well. The latter was theoretically to help the insurance funds meet the costs of medical care for unemployed or retired workers (who were no longer making contributions), and also for the care of persons with certain diseases, such as tuberculosis, which had previously been a government responsibility. The political objective of winning the favor of workers, against various socialist parties, also doubtless played a part, since the first laws were usually passed under conservative party governments.

In all countries at the outset the social insurance mechanism served essentially as a device for meeting medical expenses. It did little or nothing to change the pattern of delivery of health services. Doctors were simply paid their charges for services rendered to insured patients. To maintain fiscal solvency, a schedule of fees might have to be negotiated in advance between the insurance societies—or the government on their behalf—and representatives of the doctors, but the pattern of free choice of doctor and fee-for-service remuneration was retained. In the Scandinavian countries, in France, and in Belgium, the insurance organizations did not even pay the doctors directly. Rather, the patient paid the bill and then collected reimbursement, usually at about 80 percent of an official rate, from his insurance society. The 20 percent cost sharing by the patient was intended to discourage excessive utilization, as well as to reduce the drain on the insurance funds. There has been and continues to be much debate about the effectiveness and equity of these cost-sharing requirements. After all, it is the doctor, rather than the patient, who makes the decision on most medical services rendered. Moreover, co-payments obviously have differential impacts on families of different income levels.

As noted earlier, hospitals were not initially paid by the insurance programs, since they had evolved historically as charitable or governmental institutions. After the turn of the twentieth century, when the value of hospitalization for treatment of serious illness became greater and more widely appreciated, the insurance funds began to pay hospitals, thereby enabling them to provide better accommodations for insured patients. Medical specialists, as distinguished from general practitioners, were closely identified with hospitals in most European countries. By increasing hospital income, the insurance payments accelerated the movement, which was occurring anyway, to pay hospital specialists by salary rather than by honoraria for serving the poor. Thus, today in most of Europe specialists are usually employed by hospitals on full-time or part-time salaries for their services to insured patients, who are the great majority. A small percentage of beds may be reserved for private patients, who pay the specialist a separate private fee. Also, the part-time hospital specialist may maintain an outside office in which he sees private patients for fees.

In some countries, such as Sweden, hospitals are paid only a small share of their costs by the insurance funds, the larger part coming from local general revenues. This became the case also in Great Britain after the inauguration of its National Health Service of 1948. The British health insurance program, enacted first in 1911, was the major exception to the earlier generalization about European social insurance simply paying doctor bills according to traditional patterns. British doctors were concerned about certain of their colleagues giving excessive services and therefore being paid an unduly large piece of the financial pie allocated to a local insurance society. Therefore, by a vote of the British doctors themselves, the general practitioners decided in favor of a capitation system of remuneration. Under this system, every insured worker (dependents were not covered in the 1911 law) chose a general practitioner (GP), who was then paid a fixed monthly sum per capita for each worker on his list or panel. The GP was chosen freely by the worker, and if a worker decided to shift to another GP, his capitation payment was likewise transferred the next month. The doctor's income depended, therefore, on the number of workers he attracted to his panel, not on the number of services he rendered. His incentive for giving diligent services, of course, was to earn a reputation that would attract a maximum number of people to his panel and minimize transfers away. This capitation system for general practitioners has been continued under the comprehensive National Health Service launched in Britain in 1948.

The general trend in all the European social insurance programs, as in the earlier voluntary societies, has been to widen both the population coverage and the scope of medical services. The income threshold for mandatory coverage has been gradually raised, and additional categories of people, such as agricultural workers and even self-employed farmers and shopkeepers, have been encompassed. Services have been extended to include dental care, physiotherapy, eyeglasses, and more extensive components of institutional care, including the services of long-term nursing homes. Many preventive services, originally excluded as the province of ministries of health, have become included as benefits. Administration has become more streamlined, with consolidation of numerous small insurance societies into larger more efficient entities and development of unified systems of insurance premium collection from employers and workers. In some countries such as France and Norway, multiple independent insurance societies were converted into local offices of an integrated national system.

Most Western European countries, however, still do not protect 100 percent of their populations with social insurance for medical costs. The eligibility rules still exclude 10 or 15 percent in France, Germany, Italy, Belgium, Greece, Spain, and elsewhere, although these people may be insured voluntarily. Norway and Sweden extended their systems to every resident in the 1950's, as Great Britain had done in 1948. Eastern Europe, with socialist governments, uses other approaches that we will discuss later, but first we should see how social insurance was adopted outside of Europe.

The first non-European country to apply the social insurance approach to medical care was Japan in 1921. As in many industrial and cultural affairs, Japan emulated Germany and mandated protection of industrial workers in enterprises with five or more employees through local insurance funds. Farmers, other self-employed workers, workers in small shops, and other occupational groups did not have to be insured until another law was passed after World War II. Today about 99 percent of the Japanese population are insured, with fees paid directly by the funds to the doctor or hospital. For dependents, however, the insurance program pays only about 50 percent of the official fee, and the patient must personally pay the balance.

In 1924 Chile was the first really poor and underdeveloped country to enact social insurance for its industrial workers. The pattern of medical care delivery there, however, was quite different. The market for private fee-for-service medical practice was not strong, and the insurance organization—one central governmental fund rather than numerous local bodies—did not find it politically necessary to pay doctors on a fee basis. Instead, a more economical pattern was applied, by developing polyclinics with salaried doctors and allied personnel. Existing hospitals were used, but they were paid special supplements to provide better accommodations for insured workers (dependents were not covered). This system operated until 1952, when the broadened Chilean National Health Service was enacted, as will be discussed in a later section.

Brazil enacted a similar program in 1931, and over the next thirty years almost every Latin American country passed social insurance legislation. Since only a minor proportion of these populations were employed in industry, however, typically only a small fraction of the national population, about 10 to 15 percent, was affected. Peru passed its law in 1936, and in 1939 it established a new policy regarding hospital care. Since the existing Peruvian hospitals were relatively old and poorly designed and staffed, the National Institute for Social Security decided to build a modern new hospital in Lima exclusively for insured workers. Soon other Workers' Hospitals were built elsewhere in Peru, wherever there was a large enough number of insured people.

The Peruvian pattern was soon emulated by all the other Latin American countries enacting social security laws. Separate networks of hospitals for socially insured people were developed in almost every country of Latin America. Typically these hospitals, having greater financial support, were much better equipped and staffed than the hospitals of the ministries of health or the *beneficencia* societies. When, as in Europe, higher income (typically white collar) employees were brought under social security protection, still other national agencies were established to administer the programs. Similarly, separate networks of even higher quality hospitals were constructed for them. In Brazil, there came to be as many as seven separate social security organizations, each operating its own network of hospitals and polyclinics for different occupational classes of people.

Another special adjustment was made when higher income employees were brought under social security systems. In several Latin American countries, these middle-class persons were permitted two patterns for obtaining doctor's care. They could go to one of the polyclinics or health centers operated by their organization if they wished. They were also free to visit private doctors, and the social security fund would pay part of the fees, the balance being an obligation of the individual. This dual-choice system helped to satisfy the wishes of both the private doctors and the more affluent patients.

The Latin American social insurance systems originating later in the 1950s were less likely to establish multiple programs for different social classes. And in the 1960s there was a tendency for the multiple systems in a country, for example, in Brazil and Peru, to become coordinated or even fully integrated under one administration.

Some of the more economically developed countries of the Middle East, Iran and Turkey, for example, developed social insurance programs for medical care of regularly employed workers in the 1950s along the same lines as the Latin American countries. For similar reasons, these programs also covered only small fractions of the population, and their separate health facilities were much more technically advanced than those serving the majority of the people. Government employees were an important component of the insured persons. In Palestine, later in Israel, a unique program developed, in that it was under the control of the Federation of Labor, rather than the government. Despite this voluntary sponsorship, the pattern of delivery of care was through salaried doctors in the organization's own facilities, rather than through private resources.

India and Tunisia, also launching social security programs in this period for small portions of their populations, implemented still another approach. Instead of developing independent systems, the monies derived from contributions of workers and their employers were used to "purchase" special services from the ministries of health in those countries. With these additional funds, the ministries could build more facilities and engage health personnel to give better services to the insured persons. There were obvious administrative economies in this use of social insurance financing for strengthening the government's principal health care system, rather than developing a separate and parallel system.

In 1939 New Zealand was the first country outside the socialist world to launch a social security program that from the outset covered 100 percent of its population. Unlike the original European pattern, the program did not depend for its administration on local insurance societies but was made a direct responsibility of the national Ministry of Health and its local branches. General practitioners were paid on a fee basis, with some co-payment required from the patient. Specialist medical and surgical services, however, were given by salaried specialists in governmental hospitals without any cost sharing.

Australia was also unusual in starting its social insurance program with centrally administered pharmaceutical benefits in 1950. Gradually the list of drugs paid for was broadened from costly life-saving products to practically all the prescribed drugs used in medical practice. Then Australia adopted a strategy that has been frequently advocated in the United States. Since voluntary health insurance organizations on the model of the American "Blue" plans had developed extensively, Australia enacted legislation to encourage membership in these organizations by government subsidies. Thus, for a person enrolled in one of the approximately 90 private health insurance organizations, the reimbursement received for physician bills or the direct payment made to the hospital for in-patient care was derived in large part from government subsidies to the insurance organization. Noninsured persons did not get the benefit of these subsidies, which came from both state and federal government levels. Nevertheless, the patient still had to pay a portion of the doctor's bill. As medical fees rose, the portion payable by the patient went up, many persons remained uninsured, and difficulties developed in meeting hospital costs. Therefore, when a change of government occurred in Australia in 1972, the program was modified to a fully governmental one, covering the entire population through social insurance.

Canada and the United States were the last countries to apply the social insurance approach to financing health services on a large scale. In 1947 the province of Saskatchewan in Canada broke the ice by enacting hospitalization insurance for its whole population of about 1 million. Everyone was required to pay an earmarked hospital tax or contribution, but this was matched by an approx-imately equal allocation from provincial general revenues. The program proved so popular with the people, the hospitals, and the doctors that soon a second province (out of Canada's ten) followed suit, and by 1957 equivalent action was taken at the national level. The federal law specifies that the Canadian govern-ment will support with about 50 percent from federal revenues the cost of any provincial hospital insurance program meeting certain standards (such as covering over 95 percent of the population, paying for all general hospital care, etc.).

In 1962 Saskatchewan again pioneered the application of social insurance to the cost of physician services everywhere: office, home, and hospital. Al-though this led to a strike by the doctors, the strike was settled in three weeks by allowing several methods of medical payment (including one in which the doctor could charge the patient something extra beyond the official fee schedule). Despite this controversy, the idea proved so popular that by 1968 Canada had again enacted a national law, providing for 50 percent federal subsidy of any approved provincial program. By 1971 all ten Canadian provinces had social insurance for both hospital and physician's services, although the administrative arrangements varied.

After a long saga of legislative debate (going back to 1939), the United States enacted its Medicare law in 1965 to provide social insurance for hospital and physician's care of the aged (persons of 65 years and over drawing social security pensions). Later the totally disabled were included. The financial mechanisms differ for the hospital services, which are supported entirely from the Social Security trust fund, and the medical services, which require monthly contributions by the aged themselves and are subsidized by large allocations from federal revenues. The federal Social Security Administration is responsible for the whole program, but the handling of payments to hospitals and doctors is delegated to local voluntary insurance plans (as fiscal intermediaries). Cost sharing is also required from the aged patient. Despite its various restrictions, Medicare has led to considerably higher rates of use of hospital and medical services by old people who do, of course, have greater burdens of illness (and generally weaker financial resources) than the young.

It may be noted that many of these national systems of social security for medical care are not purely insurance but also get funds from general revenues. By being defined as social insurance, however, and getting most or a large share of their funds from earmarked contributions, they acquire certain important political advantages. Most important is stability. Since the source of funds is largely separate from that of the government as a whole, the expenditures are not subject to political debate and all the vicissitudes of the political process. Monies derived from the economic dynamics of wages and entrepreneurial earnings have an independent flow that is not competitive with the revenue demands of the numerous ministries or departments of government. Second, since the beneficiaries (workers and their dependents) themselves pay, they earn a certain entitlement of "right" to use of the money, as distinguished from the paternalistic atmosphere of charity or even governmental assistance. By the same token, the contributors of the monies—both workers and employers—are recognized to have the claim to a voice in how the monies are spent. Third, the amplitude of social insurance contributions varies directly with the strength of the whole economy; if productivity is high, social insurance income automatically increases, and vice versa, without the uncertainties of political policy changes over time.

All these attributes of social insurance are accurate only up to a point—that is, the whole social insurance mechanism depends fundamentally on legislation, and laws can be changed. However, the great attraction of the strategy, which has led to its adoption for financing health services in some seventy countries, has been its relative political stability and, in a sense, its independence from the general controversies of government. Perhaps the other side of the same coin is that the funds to support social insurance programs, being raised separately, do not impose a burden or make claims on the principal revenue sources of government from taxes on personal income, land, sales, imports, or the like. In terms of political philosophy, social insurance does not tax the rich most heavily but is fundamentally a conservative way of raising money.

General Revenues

In spite of the advantageous stability of social insurance, in contrast to other methods of financing health services, one can discern a trend in the world for mature systems of social insurance to evolve toward patterns of more and more general revenue financing. In several countries, although certainly not all, when a social insurance system becomes so well established that no political party would dare to terminate it, there has been a tendency to shift the costs increasingly or wholly to general revenues.

Perhaps the most dramatic illustration of such a cost shift was in Great Britain, where health insurance for industrial workers (not their dependents) for rather limited benefits (general practitioner care and prescribed drugs) had been operating since 1911. Then after World War II the concept of government responsibility for medical care (including the wartime program for hospitalization of casualties among civilians as well as military personnel) was so well established that in 1946 the British National Health Service law was enacted to take effect in 1948. The NHS did not eliminate social insurance funding entirely; it draws about 15 percent of its funds from this source. However, about 80 percent of the costs are derived from general revenues. (The balance of 5 percent comes from private fees.)

In 1952 Chile took somewhat similar action and, in establishing its National Health Service (covering about 70 percent of the population), drew most of its support from the general treasury, while continuing the social insurance contributions that had started in 1924. Around 1970 New Zealand shifted its financial basis form the earmarked social insurance mechanism that had started in 1939 to general revenues. Norway took similar action in 1972.

Even in the Soviet Union, the social insurance source of funds used initially to finance urban health services continued for many years after the 1917 revolution, although general government revenues were used to support health care for the large rural population. Only in 1937 were the two systems united and the whole Soviet health service put under the sphere of general revenue financing. Today, not only all personal health service—curative and preventive—but also all health facility construction, professional education, and medical research are supported by general revenues in the Soviet health system. Similar evolutions occurred in other socialist countries of eastern Europe. Also in Cuba, the voluntary *mutualista* insurance health programs were continued for many years after the 1959 revolution. Not until about 1970 was the whole Cuban health service brought under unified general revenue financing. In the People's Republic of China, this evolutionary process is currently going on, and health care at present is being financed by a great variety of local compulsory or voluntary insurance programs as well as by some private payments.

For certain sectors of the population or certain types of health service, the costs in most countries have long been borne by general revenues. Centuries before the social insurance idea was originated, the medical care of the poor in ancient Greek city-states was provided by official medical officers paid by the local government from general tax funds. After the Middle Ages, when religious charity had prevailed, local tax funds were again used for health care of the poor. The Elizabethan Poor Laws in England (around 1600) and equivalent laws in other European countries placed the responsibilities on local government to care for the "worthy poor" who were local residents. Many years later, higher levels of government contributed to the tax support—first the states or provinces in federated countries, then the national authorities. In the United States, the federal government did not contribute to the costs of medical care of the poor until 1934 (the Federal Emergency Relief Administration).

In many European countries, as noted earlier, the contribution of a government revenue share to social security programs was specifically for the purpose of supporting health services to the unemployed or indigent through the same insurance societies that paid for the care of employed workers. In the developing countries, substantial shares of the monies from central government sources to support the various ministries of health are used to finance public hospitals and health centers for serving the needs of the poor. In Africa and Asia, this usually means the majority of the population, although the magnitude of this tax support is typically much below the level of needs. Still, as education and the expectations of the people have extended, the revenue funds devoted to medical care of the poor have increased. In general, one can see a correlation between the over-all per capita wealth of a country and the amount of revenue expenditures devoted to health services for the poor.

Other population groups are also traditionally beneficiaries of health care supported by general revenues. Nearly always at the national level, this applies to the armed forces. In almost all countries, from the richest to the poorest, from the most capitalist to the most socialist, the military medical services are developed well above the level available to the general population. In numerous countries of Latin America and Africa, the military hospitals are recognized as the major centers of medical excellence. They often maintain, furthermore, special sections for civilians—members of the private power elite who pay, as well as for top officials of government outside the military services. In the United States, it is widely known that leading members of the president's cabinet or the president himself, as well as members of Congress, are often treated for their personal ailments in the Walter Reed Army Hospital or the Naval Medical Center in Washington, D.C., generally at the taxpayer's expense.

Military veterans in many countries are also often entitled to certain medical services supported by general revenues. Usually this is for disorders connected with military service, but in the United States in the absence of national health insurance for the general population veteran benefits have been extended to any type of disorder if private care would constitute a financial hardship. Other special beneficiaries of general tax-supported medical services in some countries are the original inhabitants of a territory, such as the aborigines in Australia, the Eskimos in Canada, or the Indians in the United States.

The care of persons with diseases deemed to constitute a general threat to the community, as well as being costly, is also often supported from general revenues. Serious mental disorder believed to require hospitalization (and the threshold for this judgment differs widely among countries) is probably the most widespread example. Almost all countries maintain large mental hospitals at government expense. Because of more popular competing demands for tax funds, even within the health service sector, the support for such institutions is typically very meagre, and the conditions of most mental hospitals are correspondingly poor. In many of the more affluent countries, such as Great Britain, France, and the United States, this has led to a shift in the institutional care of mental patients to general hospitals, with funding by health insurance programs.

The hospital care of tuberculosis and leprosy is also usually through general revenue funds, in the interest of protecting the population from contagion. Outside of hospitals, this system applies often to the treatment of venereal diseases in clinics or health centers. In Canada, Norway, and a few other countries, the treatment of cancer has been made a public responsibility, financed by general tax funds.

Last, and all-too-often lowest in the volume of money spent, are the general preventive health services supported by tax funds. In the developing and mainly tropical countries there are national governmental campaigns against malaria, schistosomiasis, filariasis, cholera, and other infectious diseases requiring environmental control measures. Smallpox, diphtheria, and more recently measles stimulate public immunization movements. Preventive services, consisting largely of personal health counseling to expectant mothers and small children, are offered in tax-financed clinics or health stations throughout the world. The many voluntary societies furnishing child health services typically get the bulk of their support from governmental revenue sources. Family planning, both through education and provision of contraceptive devices, is promoted mainly through tax-supported clinic programs (although the affluent usually get such services from private doctors at personal expense). Screening tests for noncommunicable diseases and health education on healthful personal behavior are other modalities of prevention usually supported by public revenues, although other economic mechanisms also play a part.

The enormous range of activities involved in sanitation and maintenance of environmental quality cannot all necessarily be defined as health services. In every country, however, the *surveillance* of water supplies, waste disposal, atmospheric purity, hygienic housing, and so on is a continuing task of governmental agencies financed by general revenues at several levels. Much of environmental health work is basically regulatory, whereas the engineering or construction aspects must be financed in a variety of ways.

Finally, foreign aid to a country for health purposes, from either international or bilateral sources, comes ultimately from general revenues of the donor nation.

This has been a very sketchy account of the medical services for the poor and of the preventive and other types of health services financed by general revenues in virtually all countries. Other forms of financing may also support many of these services, depending on the political and economic setting. The socialist countries have, in general, given a high priority to preventive services and the care of children. In general, the more industrialized and urbanized nations have invested more tax funds in the maintenance of a sanitary environment and the care of the aged.

General tax funds, or what economists define as the "public sector," are subject to great fluctuations in the amounts available for health purposes from year to year. The demands of military expenditures, the general level of prosperity, countless competing political issues—all affect the volume and adequacy of monies for the health functions reviewed in this chapter. At the same time, the very social visibility of tax-supported health programs generates pressures to assure that the money is wisely spent. If benefits are achieved and recognized, political forces tend to compel the continuation of these expenditures. It is perhaps for this reason that the long-term trend in most countries is that rising portions of a nation's wealth are being devoted to health services, and that an increasing share of these expenditures is coming from public revenues and other socially generated sources.

Readings

Andreopoulos, Spiros, (ed.), *National Health Insurance: Can We Learn from Canada?*, New York: John Wiley and Sons, 1975.

Bastos, M. V., "Brazil's Multiple Social Insurance Programs and Their Influence on Medical Care," *International Journal of Health Services, 1*:378-389 (1971).

Bridgman, R. F., "Medical Care under Social Security in France," *International Journal of Health Services, 1*:331-341 (1971).

Charron, Kenneth C., *Health Services, Health Insurance, and Their Inter-Relationships: A Study of Selected Countries*, Ottowa: Department of National Health and Welfare, 1963.

Fraser, R. D., "An International Study of Health and General Systems of Financing Health Care," *International Journal of Health Services, 3*:369-397 (1973).

Fuchs, Victor, *Who Shall Live?*, New York: Basic Books, 1974.

Glaser, William A., *Paying the Doctor: Systems of Remuneration and Their Effects,* Baltimore: Johns Hopkins Press, 1970.

Halevi, H. S., "Health Services in Israel: Their Organization, Utilization, and Finances," *Medical Care, 2*:231-242 (October-December 1964).

Hu, Tek-wei, "The Financing and the Economic Efficiency of Rural Health Services in the People's Republic of China," *International Journal of Health Services, 6*:239-250 (1976).

International Labour Office, *The Cost of Medical Care,* Geneva: ILO, 1959.

International Labour Office, *The Cost of Social Security,* Geneva: ILO, 1949-1963.

International Social Security Association, *Sickness Insurance: National Monographs,* Geneva, ISSA, 1956.

Jacobson, Charles, "The Danish Health Insurance System," *Danish Medical Bulletin, 9*:214-220 (November 1962).

Kiikuni, K., "Health Insurance Programs in Japan," *Inquiry, 9*:16-23 (March 1972).

Peters, R. J., "Health and Social Security—Some International Comparisons," in *Health Service Administration,* R. J. Peters and J. Kinnaird (eds.), Edinburgh: Livingstone, 1965, pp. 90-144.

Peterson, Osler L. et al., "What Is Value for Money in Medical Care? Experiences in England and Wales, Sweden, and the U.S.A.," *The Lancet,* 8 April 1967, pp. 771-776.

Pflanz, Manfred, "German Health Insurance: The Evolution and Current Problems of the Pioneer System," *International Journal of Health Services, 1*:315-330 (1971).

Purola, T. et al., "National Health Insurance in Finland: Its Impact and Evaluation," *International Journal of Health Services, 3*:69-88 (1973).

Roemer, Milton I., *The Organization of Medical Care under Social Security: A Study Based on the Experience of Eight Countries,* Geneva: International Labour Office, 1969.

——, "Social Security for Medical Care: Is It Justified in Developing Countries?" *International Journal of Health Services, 1*:354-361 (1971).

——, "Health Care Financing and Delivery Around the World," *American Journal of Nursing, 71*:1158-1163 (June 1971).

Roemer, Milton I. and Nobuo Maeda, "Does Social Security for Medical Care Weaken Public Health Programs?" *International Journal of Health Services, 6*:69-78 (1976).

Sigerist, Henry E., "From Bismarck to Beveridge: Development and Trends in Social Security Legislation," *Bulletin of the History of Medicine, 8*:365-388 (April 1943).

Titmuss, Richard, *The Gift Relationship,* New York: Pantheon Books, 1971.

U.S. Social Security Administration, *Social Security Programs Throughout the World, 1973,* Washington, D.C.: Government Printing Office, 1974.

Van Langendonck, J., "Social Health Insurance in the Six Countries of the European Economic Community," *International Journal of Health Services, 2*:491-502 (1972).

Wen, Chi-Pang and C. W. Hayes, "Health Care Financing in China," *Medical Care*, *14*: 241-254 (March 1976).

Winslow, C.-E. A., *The Cost of Sickness and the Price of Health*, Geneva: World Health Organization, 1951.

Wolfe, Samuel and Robin Badgley, "How Much is Enough? The Payment of Doctors—Implications for Health Policy in Canada," *International Journal Of Health Services, 4*: 245-264 (1974).

World Health Organization, *Inter-relationships Between Health Programmes and Socio-Economic Development*, Geneva: WHO Public Health Papers No. 49, 1973.

3

HEALTH MANPOWER: THE DOCTOR

In all countries, health manpower of appropriate types, in adequate numbers, and with reasonable distribution in relation to population needs is necessary to apply the knowledge of the health sciences. In this chapter we will start with a brief overview of the current health manpower landscape. Then we will focus our examination on the historically oldest practitioner of the healing arts: the doctor. First, it will provide perspective to review the history not of medical knowledge but of the doctor as the applier of that knowledge. Then we will summarize the supply (numbers) of doctors in relation to the population of different countries, the trends in this supply, and the distribution of doctors between urban and rural areas. Specialization is an important feature of medical practice, particularly in the past century, and this will be analyzed. Since the Renaissance, doctors have been prepared in medical schools; we will consider them next. Finally, we will look at associations of doctors, their role in influencing medical performance, and the difficult question of the proper supply of doctors to meet social needs.

Current Overview

Numerous types of health professions and occupations are found in every country to apply medical technology to the needs of patients. In wealthy and industrialized countries, the fields are more varied and complicated than in poorer and mainly agricultural countries, but everywhere there is the doctor of medicine who is the person most thoroughly trained to diagnose and treat the sick. Medicine has become subdivided into numerous specialties for different organ systems (e.g., opthalmology or neurology) or techniques (e.g., radiology) or demographic groups (e.g., pediatrics or gynecology), as well as general practice. In the poorer developing countries, there are also large numbers of traditional healers who until recently have had no formal education except apprenticeship and who greatly exceed the numbers of medical doctors in the rural areas.

In contrast to traditional healers, who attempt to treat every type of illness, there are various secondary practitioners, often formally trained, to whom the population have direct access for special health conditions. Among such practitioners are optometrists (in some countries called opticians) for visual refractions, podiatrists (or chiropodists) for care of superficial foot conditions, and midwives or nurse-midwives for care of pregnant women and delivery of babies. Midwives may be formally trained or they may be untrained and older village women, somewhat equivalent to the traditional healers, who are generally men. These practitioners are not to be confused with cultists (often legally recognized) who attempt to treat all disorders with one technique, such as manipulation of the spine by chiropractors.

Nurses in many, or perhaps nearly all, countries, are the most abundant type of health worker. The term "nurse" includes fully trained professional nurses, whom we will discuss later, who are often a small minority of all nurses, and large numbers of auxilliary nurses who have much less training and typically fewer educational prerequisites. Nurses' range of functions, from patient care under the doctor's orders to independent diagnosis and treatment of the common ailments (with referral of more complex cases), may be very wide, both between countries and between urban and rural districts within one country.

Auxiliary to the doctor are a wide variety of other health personnel for several special functions, more of them being found in the highly developed countries. There are technicians for laboratory examination of body fluids, excreta, or tissues. X-ray machine operation calls for radiographic or radiological technicians; even the electrocardiograph may warrant a specialized ECG technician. For various modalities in rehabilitation there are physical therapists, occupational therapists, and speech therapists. For testing hearing there may be audiologists. Auxiliary to the medical psychiatrist, there may be a psychologist and a psychiatric social worker. Similarly, a general medical social worker may assist any type of doctor in helping the patient cope with sickness and take advantage of all community resources. Moreover, ancillary to all these workers may be a second echelon of auxiliary personnel such as the laboratory assistant or the physical therapy assistant.

The handling of drugs is another special field going back to the Middle Ages. The pharmacist, modern descendant of the ancient apothecary, is the expert in identifying, storing, controlling, and dispensing an increasingly complex compendium of drugs. He has a double role—as an auxiliary to the physician (or dentist) in dispensing drugs on specific prescription (as to content, dosage, frequency and method of taking, etc.), and also as a dispenser of medications that do not legally require a doctor's order, the so-called "over-the-counter" drugs. In the latter role, especially in the poorer countries or the poorer districts of all countries, the pharmacist is often called on to give advice on the most appropriate medication.

Care of teeth, for historical reasons, has become the special province of the dentist or, in some countries, a medical specialist called stomatologist. Patients everywhere have direct access to the dentist without usually being referred by a general physician. Assisting the dentist at the chairside are various sorts of dental assistants. Doing teeth cleaning and dental health education in many countries is the dental hygienist. In an increasing number of countries, a dental nurse or dental therapist is being trained in a relatively short curriculum to give complete dental care to children. To prepare various dental prostheses or dentures (partial or complete) are dental technicians or mechanics.

With the expanding organization of health services, both curative and preventive, a whole spectrum of administrative or public health personnel have come to be necessary. These may be specialists in medicine, nursing, and other fields, or they may be wholly different types of health workers such as environmental sanitarians (sometimes called inspectors), sanitary engineers, nutritionists, health educators, or vaccinators. Health administrators may have technical competence in a clinical field or may be trained specifically for administration of hospitals, clinics, or special organized health agencies.

As new technologies develop, still further classes of health worker are trained. The inhalation therapist, a recent example, is someone skilled in the special problems of administering oxygen or special procedures for treating lung disease. The hearing aid technician, the family planning (contraception) specialist, the emergency ambulance paramedic are further types developing in response to new modalities or emphases in the health services.

With all these personnel concerned with diverse aspects of the health services, it is apparent that the individual doctor, the solo medical practitioner of old, can no longer render modern comprehensive health care by himself. A whole team of doctors, secondary practitioners, auxiliary health workers, and others is required. Even if this series of health personnel do not work together in a coordinated framework, there must be some indirect type of functional relationship among them. The demands of efficiency and effectiveness, however, are increasingly leading the many categories to work together more or less systematically, as a team in the conventional sense. The mounting recognition of the importance of prevention and therefore its closer integration with treatment, which is always more dramatically perceived, is a further pressure toward implementing the health team idea.

In this overview, we have purposely not categorized health professions as against paraprofessional personnel or health occupations. Everyone seems to agree that the doctor is the prototype of a professional person, with many implications of social independence. The status of other health personnel is the subject of much controversy, which takes different forms in different countries. In large measure, although not entirely, professional status is associated with the length of educational preparation and the freedom to make important decisions independently. Otherwise, there are arguments, both substantive and semantic, about the extent of professionalism in most other health fields. Almost all health workers seek upward social mobility, higher earnings, and greater social prestige. It is probably wisest to avoid the profession-versus-occupation argument and simply recognize that many types of personnel are needed to render comprehensive health service in any country.

History of the Doctor

Because the doctor is such a central figure in healing the sick, not to mention the oldest historically, we should look a little more into his background. The form taken by the private medical practitioner in the United States today by no means reflects all past history nor is it even representative of conditions in all countries today.

In primitive societies, the totality of health services was found in the ministrations of the medicine man or shaman. Relying on religious or magical concepts and to some extent practical experience, he invoked supernatural forces or applied physical or medicinal (herbs, minerals, etc.) means to cope with disease. In the rural areas of developing nations today, we still see a variety of indigenous healers offering mystical procedures or remedies to treat the sick. This is not to mention the Christian Scientist or "faith healer" found in sophisticated circles of many Western industrialized nations. The relationship between patient and doctor in primitive socieities is on a one-to-one basis, uncomplicated by laws or programmatic regulations, except for the influence of custom.

As society developed, social policies were formulated in laws, and some collective actions were taken to regulate health care. In ancient Babylonia, for example, most physicians were also priests, and their incantations or interpretations of omens followed theological principles. At the same time, there were nonclerical surgeons, and about 2000 B.C. the Code of Hammurabi formulated a tariff for various surgical procedures. The Code also specified punishment to the surgeon if the outcome of his efforts was poor, the severity of punishment depending on the social class of the patient.

In classical Greece, religious temples of healing were established and dedicated to the god Aesculapius, where the sick would come with offerings (one can see these votive objects in museums today) to seek miracle cures. Most Greek physicians by 500 B.C., however, had become craftsmen who, through natural observation, developed methods of diagnosis and therapy, the best known being taught by the School of Hippocrates and his followers. They traveled from town to town, setting up shop in the marketplace. In ancient Rome, the first physicians were slaves brought from Greece and attached often to large agricultural estates (*latifundia*). Later, free Greek physicians were attracted to Rome with offers of citizenship and exemption from taxes if they would settle in the towns. Greek physicians were also attached to the Roman armies as military surgeons.

With the advent of Christianity, Greek and Roman doctors came to be looked upon as practitioners of a pagan art. Most new physicians, therefore, were monks, whose practices became governed by an increasingly organized church. The monastaries had special rooms for the care of the sick, and from the sixth century onward hostels or hospitals were established for the care of the impoverished sick and destitute. By the twelfth century, however, a reaction occurred against the preoccupation of monks or priests with so worldly a matter as treatment of the patient's body. Surgery, shedding blood, was particularly unsuitable. Therefore, laymen became engaged in medicine and surgery—two rather separate fields (notice that the licensure laws of many states still designate a doctor as "physician and surgeon"). The first medical school for laymen was founded at Salerno, Italy during the ninth century, and it flourished for several hundred years. During the twelfth and thirteenth centuries, universities were established throughout Europe to educate, among others, physicians.

As the towns developed after the Renaissance, doctors educated in the universities settled in them as private practitioners. A coveted goal, however, was to become attached to a feudal estate or a royal court as a salaried body physician. In this role, the doctor would serve the noble and his family, as well as giving some assistance to the lowly serfs. At the same time in the towns was a lower class of artisans, offering for a fee such special skills as setting broken bones or extracting teeth. The barbers often did bloodletting, to release harmful "humors," and some evolved into barber-surgeons. Another occupational group, not trained by the universities and of lower social status, were the apothecaries who set up shop with all sorts of products from vegetable, animal, or mineral sources. Poor people went directly to the apothecaries for help at lower prices than those charged by doctors, as applies to pharmacists to this day. During the later Middle Ages these several occupational groups—the doctors, the barber-surgeons, the apothecaries—formed guilds to protect their trade interests, and then set standards for admission to the guilds.

With the growth of hospitals after the twelfth century, but much more rapidly with the industrialization of the eighteenth and nineteenth centuries, the character of the medical profession was further altered. Hospitals became centers of medical education, usually in association with universities, and also gave rise to specialization, not only as between medicine and surgery but within each of these disciplines. With numerous patients having similar disorders located in one hospital ward, specialization developed for the treatment of various types of hospital patient. In Europe, only the better educated and usually upper-class physicians were appointed to serve in hospitals (as an honor in a spirit of noblesse oblige to aid the poor), so that by the twentieth century two classes of doctor had developed—those attached to hospitals, who were increasingly specialized, and those practicing entirely outside hospitals as general practitioners.

With the settlement of North America in the seventeenth century, mainly by the British and French, the medical evolution that had been seen in Europe was repeated in the New World in much shorter time. The early doctors came from Europe (as the Roman doctors had come from Greece), and others were trained by apprenticeship. With no feudal estates, however, virtually all doctors set up shop as small tradesmen in the towns. The first hospital was not founded until 1750 in Philadelphia, and then small hospitals to which virtually all local doctors had access came to be built in many new towns. With less rigid classes than characterized Europe, the sharp line between hospital and community doctors did not form. To train more doctors, medical schools were formed around urban hospitals, usually unassociated with any university, so that by the end of the nineteenth century there were 160 medical schools in the United States.

By 1900 a large supply of doctors existed in America—about 1 for every 700 people, which was more than in any European country at the time. Their qualifications, of course, were quite uneven. The states had passed medical licensure laws after the Civil War, but they were relatively lax. A movement by the medical association and some philanthropic foundations began, which culminated in the important Flexner Report in 1910, leading to the closure of many substandard medical schools. With fewer medical schools, the supply of doctors declined. The increase in scientific knowledge, however, led to expansion of specialization, but not linked so closely to hospitals as in Europe. In the world scene, this independence of specialties from the hospitals was exceptional, since policies on the other continents were more influenced by European colonizers than by Americans who were "colonizing" their own land mass, as they moved their frontier from the east to the west.

A small share of doctors in America, as well as Europe, served in salaried positions with the military services, certain large hospitals, in public health agencies, and in certain isolated industries at the turn of the twentieth century. The great majority were in private medical practice. They charged fees for each type of service. In the United States these were usually paid directly by the patient, but in Europe (as we will discuss shortly) the fee payments came to be made increasingly by insurance sickness funds. Competition developed to attract patients and, as we will also discuss later, codes of medical ethics and etiquette developed to control it. The doctor in the industrialized countries developed more and more of the characteristics of a small business man, selling his wares in an open market.

In the largely impoverished colonies of the European powers in Asia, Africa, and Latin America, the history of the doctor was quite different. Except for a handful of private medical practitioners serving the prosperous in the national or provincial capitals, doctors of the nineteenth century were salaried civil servants of the colonial medical services, mainly from the mother country. The mass of the population got attention for their ailments from various auxiliary health workers, trained by apprenticeship, or from purely traditional untrained healers. As the colonies became emancipated in the twentieth century, various systems of organized health service with salaried personnel replaced the colonial systems, but at the same time with expanding middle classes a larger volume of private practice developed. More about these countries and programs will be discussed later.

In the industrialized countries, the world-wide economic depression of the 1930s had a profound impact on the patterns of practice of the doctor. Social insurance programs to support medical care costs, which had been extending gradually in Europe, spread to other continents—to Latin America, Japan, New Zealand, the Middle East. Many public programs of medical care for the poor were strengthened in America, and doctor's care for the ambulatory became organized increasingly through hospital outpatient departments, community health centers, and private group practice. The first fully socialized system of health care, with all doctors working as civil servants of the government, moved ahead in the Soviet Union and began to exert an influence on other countries, such as India.

With World War II, the concept of national planning of health services, previously identified with the socialist USSR, spread to virtually all countries. The doctor as the acknowledged leader of the health care team, came to be increasingly influenced by these trends. The private entrepreneurial character of medical practice became steadily modified by patterns of work in which doctors served within organized frameworks. The structure and function of these will be analyzed in the coming pages.

Numbers, Trends, and Distribution of Doctors

To say that there were about 2 million physicians to serve the world's 1975 population of about 4 billion (a global ratio of 1:2000) people is a rather pointless statement, but it may help us enter this jungled terrain. The point is that there are many differences in the definition and functions of a physician in various countries. It is less his numbers or even ratios to population that count than the great variations in these ratios among countries and between different regions within each country. There are numerous types of physician, as between diverse specialists and general practitioners (or more simply generalists), which we will explore later. There are varying relationships of the doctor supply to the economic level and the prevailing political ideology of each country. There are many variations in the scope of functions of the physician in relation to the functions of other personnel. The structural framework, within which the physician works (or delivers his service) is important enough to warrant separate discussion later. The trends in physician output and supply can also give us clues to the future.

Perhaps the central fact to understand is that some type of person skilled in healing the sick (prevention of disease unfortunately is still, in most countries, a secondary consideration) and having had a maximum amount of training, is found everywhere in the world. His numbers and ratio to population, however, differ enormously among countries, depending largely, but by no means entirely, on national wealth. The United States, with about 330,000 doctors for a population of 215 million has a current ratio of 1 doctor per 650 people, or about 15 doctors per 10,000 population, to put it another way. Ethiopia, at the other extreme, has about 400 doctors (many of them expatriates from other countries) to serve its 28 million people or a ratio of 1 doctor to about 70,000 persons. Thus, in terms of doctor-to-population ratios, the United States has more than 100 times the supply of doctors found in Ethiopia. The per capita wealth of the two countries in this example is roughly corresponding; the per capita gross domestic product (GDP) of the United States is about $5,400 per year, compared to about $65 per year in Ethiopia.

In between these two polar examples among the roughly 140 countries in the world there are many deviant variations. Western European countries have ratios of generally better than 1:1,000, Latin American countries vary widely between about 1:600 in Argentina (the most abundantly supplied) to 1:4,000 in Guatemala and 1:10,000 in Haiti. A line drawn on a graph setting the doctor supply against the per capita wealth of different countries would not be perfectly straight, although it would show a generally positive linear correlation. The point is that there are various other factors, outside of the economic, that also influence a nation's supply of doctors. History and political ideology play large parts, especially the latter. As a matter of political principle, the socialist countries have placed a high priority on producing doctors, and several of them, despite much lower over-all per capita incomes than the United States, have higher ratios of doctors. The Soviet Union, for example, still much less affluent than the United States, has one doctor to about 310 persons (not counting its thousands of *feldshers*, of whom we will say more later). For other reasons, the Philippine Republic, although a very poor country of many thousand islands, trains a great many doctors each year at numerous private medical schools. Although many leave the country, the Philippines retain enough to have a ratio of 1:1,500—much more than other equally poor countries of Asia.

The trend in most countries over the past century and especially since the colonial emancipations following World War II has, nevertheless, been for an increased output of doctors at rates higher than the growth of population. Toward the end of the colonial era in Africa, the British, French, and other European powers started medical schools in several capital cities; one of the first moves after national emancipation or liberation was to expand these schools and build new ones. The accelerated output of doctors has been especially great in Latin America where in 1959 a social revolution in Cuba led to a great drive to improve human welfare services in the other countries of this depressed continent. Medical schools were increased and enlarged, and despite a rapid rate of population growth (there is little family planning in these Catholic countries), the Latin American doctor-population ratio increased from 5.3 per 10,000 in 1957 to 7.4 by 1969. Similar though less dramatic increases have been achieved in other developing continents.

Along with the accelerated training of doctors there naturally occurs a greater output of other allied health personnel—not only nurses, but pharmacists, technicians, rehabilitation therapists, various types of medical assistant, and others. One of the possible explanations of the strikingly high rate of increase of doctors in Latin America has been a somewhat negative attitude toward substitute medical assistants who have been much more widely used in Asia and Africa, where colonial medical systems had been in control until much more recent times. Another likely factor has been the fairly rapid growth of social insurance systems in most Latin American countries to finance medical care for the steadily employed portions of the population, thereby providing economic support for many more doctors. This trend has not been seen to nearly the same degree in Asia or Africa. We will discuss this more fully in Chapter 4.

In spite of the substantial increases in the world's supply of doctors, their availability to serve people within any individual country has remained extremely uneven. The greatest disparities mark the doctor resources for the rural as compared with the urban populations. It is common for 75 percent or more of the doctors in a poor developing country to be located in the capital city. Tunis, for example, which has about 20 percent of the national population of Tunisia, has approximately 75 percent of the doctors. The remaining 80 percent of the people must be served mainly by the balance of 25 percent of the doctors. Even though some rural people do travel long distances to a metropolitan center for medical care, the inequity remains enormous. Various strategies, with different degrees of success, have been applied to tackle this problem.

The medical maldistribution problem is found in all countries, even in the United States and the prosperous lands of Europe. There are vast disparities among the states of the United States, with Connecticut in 1970, for example, having 17.8 active doctors per 10,000 population, compared with 8.1 per 10,000 in Arkansas. Although many cultural factors play a part, the per capita wealth of a region is obviously a major one, just as it is with nations. Within single cities, moreover, a skewed distribution in the location of doctors between fashionable neighborhoods and slum areas is the general rule. This is particularly marked for specialists whose private offices are concentrated in London's Harley Street no less than in the Beverly Hills district of Los Angeles.

Another distributional problem has become prominent in recent years as world-wide mobility has increased and many countries have relaxed their immigration restrictions. In the nineteenth century, some small movement of doctors from Europe to the colonies on other continents occurred. Dutch doctors, who found Holland medically overcrowded, went to build a new life in the Dutch East Indies (now Indonesia), enjoying at the same time some foreign adventure and the comforts of a colonial household with many servants. The same sort of movement occurred from Belgium to the Congo, from London to Bombay, from Paris to Saigon. However, in the twentieth century, and especially after the national liberations following World War II, the migrations moved mainly in the opposite direction. Indian doctors trained in Madras came to London for postgraduate study; young doctors from Cambodia or Algeria came to France, or from Djakarta to Amsterdam. When their specialized studies were over, they often stayed on, not only because of the more stimulating and lucrative life in the European cities but also because there simply were not opportunities for them to apply their newly gained knowledge in their impoverished homelands.

As the United States after World War II became increasingly the wealthiest nation in the world, it became the magnet attracting the largest numbers of medical migrants. With America's great medical centers demonstrating the very latest in technology, hundreds and even thousands of young doctors were drawn from the Philippines and Iran, from Chile and Mexico, from Turkey and Egypt. More often than not, it seemed, they never returned home. And although they seldom found openings in the famous and prestigious medical centers, they were welcomed in the sidetrack positions shunned by American medical school graduates— in the mental hospitals, the public general hospitals for the chronically ill or poor, or the smaller hospitals lacking any university affiliation. Medical migrants came also from other industrialized countries, from Great Britain and Austria, from Japan and Australia, not so much for training as for wider practice opportunities.

The "brain drain," as it came to be called (and it applied in engineering, the basic sciences, etc. as well) became a prominent issue in the 1960s and 1970s. It could not be interpreted as the United States serving as a land of refuge for the escapees from Nazi Germany, from the frustrated counterrevolution in Hungary, or from Fidel Castro's Cuba. Instead, it was thought of as the rich America taking medical resources from the poor developing lands, who needed doctors desperately and had invested in their education. The likelihood that this education was inferior to American standards was tolerated. To protect American patients the Educational Commission for Foreign Medical Graduates (ECFMG) was formed to administer an examination, and only those who passed it (usually less than half) were licensed. Despite the inequities for the home country, some spoke of the "freedom to migrate"; if something were to be done to redress the imbalances, it should come from the initiative of the home country, not the United States. In the 1970s, the problem was attracting the attention of the World Health Organization, but the answer was not clear.

Specialization

Another crucial aspect of medical practice, one that is increasingly important, is specialization. We have discussed the separate medieval origins of medicine and surgery and their coming together only in the eighteenth and nineteenth centuries. In ancient Egypt, specialized medical artisans were described by the Greek traveler and scholar, Herodotus. These early specialists were skilled in disorders of the skin, of the eyes, of trauma, of fevers, and so on. In the early towns of Europe, artisans who had no formal education developed skills at pulling teeth, setting broken bones, or even removing from the eyes cataracts that caused blindness.

Specialization as a matter for formal training, however, did not apply to the university-trained doctor until the mid-nineteenth century. The masterly physician was expected to be competent at everything. Then, with the dawn of bacteriology and cellular pathology in late nineteenth century Europe, the volume of medical knowledge became overwhelming. For many years, a doctor who was beginning to concentrate on a specialty would continue his service to other types of patient as well. Until after the turn of the twentieth century, exclusive specialization, it was feared, verged a little on charlantanism. The true physician, it was thought, was the man (rarely, indeed, the woman) of great breadth.

Well before the eighteenth century, specialized subjects were taught in the medical schools, not only anatomy (normal and morbid) and *materia medica* (pharmacology) but also surgery, obstetrics and diseases of women (gynecology), internal or clinical medicine, ophthalmology, neurology, and dermatology. However, medical practice was another matter. It was in the United States that the first declaration of exclusive dedication to specialized practice occurred. The first specialty board certification was established for ophthalmology in 1916. Nineteenth-century Vienna had doctors famed in ophthalmology and otolaryngology, but most of them were attached to hospitals and teaching institutions. When the Royal College of Physicians was established by British royal decree in 1518, it signified not specialization in internal medicine but a kind of basic medical licensure, and the establishment of the Royal College of Surgeons in 1800 served mainly to elevate the status of surgeons to that of physicians. Abraham Jacobi, who came to the United States from Germany in the mid-nineteenth century, trained a following in diseases of children (pediatrics). Reginald H. Fitz of Harvard, who first described appendicitis in 1886, helped to establish surgery of the abdomen as a field of specialization. However, specialized practice was not common until the late nineteenth or early twentieth centuries.

The growth of medical knowledge after the early twentieth century came at such a rapid pace that the whole image of the physician was bound to change. Even outside the medical schools, excellence became associated with specialization more than with generalism. After the end of World War I, in the early 1920s, the dominant voices in the American Medical Association became those of the specialists more than of the general family doctors, a fact that may account for the change of philosophical posture of the AMA at that time from liberal humanism to extreme conservatism. (A few years before 1920, the AMA had set up a committee to study health insurance; a few years after, the same concept was condemned as "alien and socialistic.") In any case, by 1920 specialization was rapidly advancing in both the United States and Europe. Various royal colleges and academies in Britain, France, and the countries under their influence began to certify competence in specialized fields. In the United States, numerous specialty boards took shape. A key feature of specialty board certification in the United States was *exclusive* dedication to one particular discipline.

In Europe and the numerous countries influenced by it, specialty practice—because of its historic association with hospitals—was closely linked to hospital appointments. Only a minority of European doctors even to the present time, have appointments to hospital staffs, at least to public hospitals where the significant work is done. (Small private hospitals may be open to any doctor for minor surgical or obstetrical work.) It is these doctors who are the specialists or consultants, although part of their time may also be spent in a private office outside the hospital.

In the United States, the relationship of doctors to hospitals was closer and of longer duration, and specialization was correspondingly more prevalent. The great majority of physicians, both specialists and generalists, became affiliated with community hospitals. Most specialized service was rendered in private offices, rather than in hospital outpatient departments. With a larger middle class of moderate or high income, the market for the higher-priced specialty services was greater, and medical specialization grew more rapidly than in any other country. From about 80 percent generalists and 20 percent specialists in 1920, the proportions reversed to about 80 percent specialists and 20 percent generalists fifty years later. Although not so extreme as in the United States, the trend to specialization has occurred in all countries, but most markedly in those that are more industrialized. Australia, for example, currently has about 55 percent specialists, and health leaders are concerned about the decline of general family doctors to 45 percent of the total.

In the 1960s a reaction set in, especially in the more industrialized countries, to strengthen the field of general practice. Much of the attraction of the specialties was the higher earning potential and professional prestige. In response, more elaborate training programs for family medicine were developed, and this field was granted a kind of specialty status backed up by royal colleges and specialty boards in many different countries. With this went higher rewards in schedules of medical fees or in salaried positions. By 1970, the pendulum was beginning to swing back toward more balanced proportions between general practice and the specialties.

Another reaction to specialization in many countries has been the training of greater numbers of middle-level health personnel who, in an organized framework, serve to screen out patients with simple ailments so as to save the time of the busy general practitioner. As noted in Chapter 1, such personnel had long been used in the colonial medical systems, in both Czarist Russia and the USSR, and in the military services of all types of country. In the United States, military corpsmen returning from the Vietnam war were trained as physician assistants, and later graduate nurses were trained as nurse practitioners. In other countries, nurses called clinical or community nurses were trained and authorized to carry out functions previously reserved for doctors. Also, nurse-midwives and nurse-anesthetists had long been practicing obstetrics and anesthesia in hospitals (as well as in homes) in many countries of Europe and elsewhere. With increasing appreciation of the psychosomatic and psychosocial aspects of disease, a fresh appreciation of the importance of "good general practice," as the British call it, has arisen everywhere. In improving the organization of general health service delivery everywhere, greater attention is being paid to the necessity that every person have access to a primary health practitioner, whether a doctor or someone less fully trained. The primary health practitioner serves as "gatekeeper" to the whole health service system, referring patients to medical specialists or to other types of health worker as necessary.

Medical Schools

The formal training of doctors in medical schools, as noted earlier, began in ninth century Italy at Salerno. A century later, while most of Europe was still in its Dark Ages, a medical school was founded at Cairo, Egypt, in 972 A.D., where ancient classical culture was, to some extent, being kept alive by Arabian scholars. Throughout the subsequent centuries, up to the sixteenth, all university training for medicine was found in the cities of Europe, including Oxford and Cambridge in England, Krakow and Rostow in the eastern Slavic regions, and Copenhagen in the north. However, it was predominantly in southern and central Europe— Italy, France, and Germany. It was not until 1551 that the first medical school was established outside Europe at Mexico City under the influence of Spain. The first medical school in the British colonies that are now the United States was founded in Boston at Harvard University in 1782 (although the university had been started as a theological seminary in 1636). Other medical faculties were organized in Latin America in Caracas, Venezuela, in 1725, Santiago, Chile, in 1743, Rio de Janeiro, Brazil, in 1808, Buenos Aires, Argentina, in 1821, and Montevideo, Uruguay, in 1840. The first medical school in English Canada (Dalhousie University) was founded in Halifax in 1818 and in French Canada (Laval University) in Quebec City in 1852. Not until 1868 was a medical school founded on any other continent—in Tokyo, Japan. Another was founded in Hong Kong by the British in 1887. The University of the Philippines, under American influence, established a medical school in 1908.

Thus it is apparent that for the most part medical schools in the world today are of relatively recent origin. A compilation of all known medical schools by the Italian medical historian, Arturo Castiglioni, up to 1922 identified 229 schools throughout the world. There may have been omissions in this listing but, on the other hand, many schools recorded no longer operate today. In 1953, the World Health Organization compiled a *World Directory of Medical Schools* as of that date and, although also admitting to probable omissions, found just over 500 institutions, or about 275 more than the listing prepared thirty years before. In other words, in the thirty years from 1923 to 1953, more medical schools were established than in the previous 1,000 years. Since 1953, the rate of medical school foundings has further accelerated. In the two decades from 1953 to 1973, for example, medical schools in the United States increased from 79 to 115, in Canada from 11 to 16, in the Philippines from 4 to 7, in Cuba from 1 to 3, and in the People's Republic of China they more than doubled from 33 to 85.

With certain important exceptions, medical schools are parts of universities. A few medical schools in the United States, however, which originated solely from the organizational base of a large hospital, are not university affiliated. On the other hand, some institutions of higher learning sponsor more than one medical school. The University of London sponsors twelve medical schools, each associated with a separate hospital, and the University of California has five, each at a different campus location in this large American state. The most important exception to the usual association of a medical school with a university, however, is in the Soviet Union where in 1937 the approximately sixty university-based medical schools were removed from their parent universities and set up as separate training and service institutes, thus being transferred from the supervision of the Ministry of Education to that of the Ministry of Health. It was considered that by this move the content of medical education and the quantitative output of doctors would be planned in closer relation to the health needs of the population, for which the Ministry of Health is responsible. This policy has been emulated in most of the other socialist countries, although not in all. In Czechoslovakia and Cuba, medical schools are still university linked.

The conventional schedule of medical education in the United States, with a four-year bachelor's degree followed by a four-year medical degree program, is the exception on the world scene. The usual schedule in Europe and elsewhere is entrance of the student directly to medical school following primary and secondary schooling, which usually consists of a total of ten to eleven years. Then the student is engaged in studies of both basic and clinical sciences for a continuous period of five to six years. Often the sixth year is essentially a hospital internship under only indirect medical school supervision, but the degree is awarded only after its completion. In the majority of countries, all or almost all applicants for training (especially in the poorer developing countries) are admitted, but large proportions fail after the first year or two. It is not unusual, as in Guatemala for example, for a medical school to admit 1,000 candidates and to graduate at the end of six years only about 300.

This open admission policy is doubtless associated with the fact that in nearly all countries the medical schools are all or almost all government controlled and financed. Here again the United States and countries heavily influenced by its private enterprise ideology (e.g., post World War II Japan and the Philippines) are the exceptions. Being tax supported, they are regarded as accessible to any student who has completed the prerequisite education; then if he does not meet academic standards, he is not allowed to continue. This public support probably also means greater standardization in the content of education, although in most countries the universities still enjoy much autonomy despite their fiscal dependence on government, and innovations within broad boundaries are not inhibited. Another implication of the public financing of most medical education throughout the world relates to licensure. Since the universities are inherently approved by a ministry of education, graduation from them is accepted as proof of adequate competence. Legal permission to engage in medical practice, or "medical registration," then simply requires proof of graduation from an approved school and perhaps an internship or other such requirement, but not a second examination by a medical licensure body.

On a world scale, the great majority of medical students are young men, just as the great majority of nursing school students are young women. With the Russian Revolution, however, this pattern suddenly changed in the USSR and then in the newer socialist countries. In these nations about 50 percent or even higher proportions of medical students are women. This has come about not only because of a deliberate policy of equal opportunity for the two sexes but also because men attending higher educational institutions have tended more often to concentrate in engineering and the basic sciences. Another factor is a policy of vertical mobility in the health occupations, which means that many medical students are drawn from former nurses or *feldshers* (medical assistants). A similar tendency to train rising proportions of women in medicine is now seen also in India, Brazil, the United States, and other nonsocialist countries.

Medical education in the Soviet Union and in other socialist countries influenced by the USSR differs also in other respects. In most of the Soviet medical schools there are three basic curriculum tracks: general medicine, pediatrics, and hygiene. The first two years are the same for all students, but then he or she must make a choice among the three paths. The majority choose general medicine or "therapeutics." The second most popular choice is pediatrics, which attracts women almost entirely; the remainder (only 5 to 10 percent) take the hygiene path. A much greater emphasis is given to hygiene and social medicine in all three Soviet medical school tracks, however, than in the schools of other nations. Similarly, in Latin America and Africa, preventive and social medicine tend to receive much more attention in the medical schools than in North America or Europe.

The People's Republic of China recently startled Western observers by shortening its course for medical studies from six years to three or three-and-a-half. The objective is to greatly accelerate the output of doctors and to emphasize practical training in the management of the highly prevalent diseases, along with prevention, with less attention to theoretical instruction in the basic sciences. Whether this policy will continue after China trains enough doctors to meet the needs of its huge population (750 million or more) remains to be seen. In American medical education there has also been a recent, although less radical, tendency to shorten the years of medical training by introducing more elective course time at an early stage to shorten the eventual period required for qualifying in a specialty.

The great turning point in medical education in the United States came in 1910, when the national survey of schools culminating in the Flexner Report led to a sharp up-grading of academic standards, especially in stressing the need for full-time teachers for both basic and clinical sciences. Through establishing a system of grading medical schools as A, B, or C, the policies of state licensure boards and the forces of the free market soon led to the closing of all except the grade A schools. The influence of Flexner, whose background was German scholarship, was to put great emphasis on the basic sciences and on technical procedures, perhaps at the expense of the humanistic or social aspects of medicine. This contributed, perhaps, to the enormous acceleration of specialization in the United States. American medical schools, in turn, influenced teaching patterns in other countries, especially after World War II.

In one respect, however, the medical schools of the poorer developing countries have not been able to emulate an American model: They have been unable to engage full-time faculty members. To pay adequate salaries to support full-time medical professors is very expensive, so that few schools in Latin America, Asia, or Africa have such teachers. Nearly all medical school professors on these continents also engage in private practice—typically serving the very affluent—to earn a satisfactory, often high, income. This tends to impair the quality of medical education in most of the developing countries.

Medical Societies, Ethics, and Needs

When competition among private doctors became a prominent feature of medical practice in the eighteenth and nineteenth centuries, various commercialized practices developed to attract patients. Most prominent was advertising, often with extravagant claims about a doctor's ability to cure various ailments. There was also price competition, and when a patient was attracted to a doctor charging lower fees he was often greeted with derogatory comments about the previous doctor's service.

In the early nineteenth century, doctors of the more industrialized countries began to form medical societies that, among other things, established standards to guide the behavior of their members. The British Medical Association was founded in 1832. The BMA is not to be confused with the Royal Colleges of Physicians and of Surgeons established by the monarch's decree much earlier essentially as licensing bodies. In 1845 the French Society of Medicine was founded and in 1847 the American Medical Association. Much later equivalent associations of doctors were formed in other countries. These associations typically conducted educational programs for their members, but more important were their efforts to promulgate what other occupations might call "fair trade practices." These efforts were associated with exerting an influence on medical education, selectivity in granting doctors membership in the association, and outright opposition to quackery or medical cultism.

One of the special contributions of the medical associations was formulation of codes of ethics, which were really mixtures of ethical guides on the doctor's obligations to his patient and rules of etiquette for the doctor's behavior in relation to other doctors. In England, Sir Thomas Percival published in 1803 a seminal Code of Medical Ethics, which proposed various rules for the doctor's conduct ranging from personal temperance to respecting the confidence of the patient and not speaking in a loud voice on the hospital ward. The Oath of Hippocrates, attributed to the ancient Greek master, had been used as a ceremonial oath for new medical school graduates for centuries in Europe and was primarily a promise of allegiance by the student to his teacher. It was also an affirmation that he would behave with integrity toward his patients, respecting their secrets and doing no harm—including refraining from "fornication with woman or man" among his patients (the very presence of such a declaration in the oath suggests that it was a problem).

These codes and oaths were not a matter of law (although some of their principles later became embodied in medical practice statutes), but they exerted a disciplinary influence on medical practice in an expanding competitive industrial society. The American Medical Association, in its founding, was motivated largely by opposition to quackery and advertising, which were rampant in the young American society at the time. The upgrading of United States medical schools at the opening of the twentieth century was in no small measure due to the leadership of the AMA. In addition, specialty societies in surgery, ophthalmology, pathology, pharmacology, public health, and other disciplines were founded principally to advance knowledge and exchange of ideas in these fields.

As governments exerted an increasing influence on the financial support of medical care, especially after the birth of social insurance in Germany in the 1880s, the medical associations came to play another role. Since most doctors did not work for wages, they did not form trade unions, but the medical associations performed a similar function in bargaining with governments or with various sickness insurance funds regarding the fees that would be paid for designated services. Schedules of fees were published by medical societies, to encourage fair prices that ought to be charged by their members (hence, reducing price competition), as well as to serve as a basis for bargaining with governments and other third-party payers. Although such price-fixing in other enterprises was deemed illegal under the U.S. Sherman Anti-Trust Act of 1890, medical service at the time was not considered a trade, and their policy was calmly accepted.

Every European country had its medical association by the end of the nineteenth century, and by about 1920 almost every sovereign nation in the world had an equivalent society. The colonies often formed branches of the medical association in the mother country, as did the associated semiautonomous countries in the British or French groupings of nations—for example, the Australian Branch of the British Medical Association. With the accelerated extension of governmental programs of medical care, these associations acquired increasingly an adversary posture to protect the business interests of the private physician against the inroads of government. In the United States, the medical associations in the states and counties, as well as nationally, saw themselves as defenders of traditional patterns of medical practice. Even without governmental involvement, they opposed and often declared "unethical" doctors' innovative methods. Thus, even private group medical practice, with or without associated voluntary insurance for patients, was condemned as unethical and was opposed in various ways.

In countries where economic development yielded a relatively large market for private practice, one of the other important effects of medical societies was to exert an effect on the total output of physicians. Through indirect influence on the enrollments in medical schools and more direct influence on the passing of examinations for various specialty societies, doctors could limit the numbers of their competitors. This influence was especially keenly felt during the worldwide economic Depression of the 1930s when in relation to reduced purchasing power the medical profession appeared to be overcrowded. As a result, the training of additional physicians was inhibited, and in the 1950s and 1960s, when economic support for medical care was much expanded, shortages of doctors were felt in many countries.

After the end of World War II in 1945, the output of doctors in most countries was steadily increased. Questions were repeatedly raised about the "correct supply" of physicians to meet a population's health needs. The answer obviously depends on many factors. Among them are: (1) the money available to finance medical care, (2) the means of remuneration of doctors, whether by fees, salaries, capitation, or other methods, (3) the patterns of medical practice, especially with respect to the use of ancillary personnel, (4) the rate of demand for medical service, which in turn is influenced by levels of education, transportation, epidemiological factors, cultural or behavior traits, and so on, (5) the incentives in the medical care system, since most medical services are generated by decisions of the doctor rather than the patient, (6) the effectiveness of disease prevention or health promotion, and so on. We have noted that some countries, such as the Soviet Union or Israel, have about 1 doctor to 400 people, and still believe they need more. Others, India, for example, have 1 doctor to 5,000 or 6,000 people, and yet many of those trained leave the country because they cannot find remunerative work to do.

The correct supply of doctors, therefore, must depend on the economic and the social policy characteristics of the whole health care system, and also on the supply and functions of many other types of health personnel. We will examine in later pages, the configuration of total health care systems but in the next section we will look briefly at the main features in different countries of other members of the health care team who work with the doctor.

Readings

Association of American Medical Colleges, *Study of Community Health Training Programs in Schools of Medicine in Four Selected Developing Countries,* Washington, D.C., October 1974.

Badgley, Robin and Samuel Wolfe, *Doctors' Strike: Medical Care and Conflict in Saskatchewan,* New York: Atherton Press, 1967.

Blishen, B. R., *Doctors and Doctrines,* Toronto: University of Toronto Press, 1969.

Bowers, J. Z. and E. Purcell (eds.), *National Health Services, Their Impact on Medical Education and Their Role in Prevention,* New York: Josiah Macy, Jr. Foundation, 1973.

Bunker, J. P., "Surgical Manpower: A Comparison of Operations and Surgeons in the United States and in England and Wales," *New England Journal of Medicine, 282*:135-144 (1970).

Butler, Irene, "The Migratory Flow of Doctors to and from the United States," *Medical Care, 9*:17-31 (January-February 1971).

Colombian Ministry of Public Health and Colombian Association of Medical Schools, *Study on Health Manpower and Medical Education in Colombia, Vol. II, Preliminary Findings,* Washington, D.C.: Pan American Health Organization, 1967.

Dimond, E. Grey, "Medical Education and Care in the People's Republic of China," *Journal of the American Medical Association, 218*:1552-1557, 6 December 1971.

Fein, Rashi, *The Doctor Shortage: An Economic Diagnosis,* Washington, D.C.: Brookings Institution, 1967.

Forsyth, Gordon, *Doctors and State Medicine,* Philadelphia: Lippincott Co., 1966.

Garcia, Juan Cesar, "Profile of Medical Education in Latin America," *International Journal of Health Services, 1*:37-59 (1971).

Gish, Oscar (ed.), *Doctor Migration and World Health: The Impact of the International Demand for Doctors on Health Services in Developing Countries,* London: G. Bell and Sons, 1971.

Hall, Thomas L., *Health Manpower in Peru,* Baltimore: Johns Hopkins Press, 1969.

Hogarth, J., *The Payment of Physicians: Some European Comparisons,* New York: Free Press, 1963.

Leake, Chauncey D. (ed.), *Percival's Medical Ethics,* Baltimore: Williams and Wilkins Co., 1927.

Leon, C. A., "Psychiatry in Latin America," *British Journal of Psychiatry, 125*: 121-136 (August 1972).

Mann, K. J., "The Israel Physician: His Training, Responsibilities and Rights," *Israel Journal of Medical Science, 6*:145-153 (January-February 1970).

Omran, A. R. (ed.), *Community Medicine in Developing Countries,* New York: Springer Publishing Co., 1974.

Otsyula, W., "Native and Western Healing: The Dilemma of East African Psychiatry," *Journal of Nervous and Mental Disorders, 156*:297-299 (May 1973).

Poffenbarger, P. L., "Physicians in South Vietnam—Controversies and Needs," *New England Journal of Medicine, 284*:1065-1071 (May 1971).

Purcell, Elizabeth (ed.), *World Trends in Medical Education, Faculty, Student, and Curriculum,* Baltimore: Johns Hopkins Press, 1971.

Rexed, Bror, "The Role of Medical Education in Planning the Development of a National Health Care System," *Journal of Medical Education, 49*:27-42 (January 1974).

Rozer, F., "Doctor for Newly Developed Nations," *Journal of Medical Education, 35*:918-924 (October 1964).

Sigerist, Henry E., "Medical Societies, Past and Present," *Yale Journal of Biology and Medicine, 6*:351-362 (January 1934).

——, *Medicine and Human Welfare,* New Haven: Yale University Press, 1941, Chap. III.

——, "The Place of the Physician in Modern Society," *Proceedings of the American Philosophical Society, 90*:275-279 (September 1946).

Southall, Roger J., "The Politics of Medical Higher Education in East Africa," *Social Science and Medicine, 6*:413-424 (June 1972).

Waldenstrom, "The Social and Economic Situation of the Medical Profession in Sweden," *New England Journal of Medicine, 221*:515-518 (1939).

Williams, Kathleen N. and Betty A. Lockett, "Migration of Foreign Physicians to the United States: The Perspective of Health Manpower Planning," *International Journal of Health Services, 4*:213-243 (1974).

World Health Organization, *World Health Statistics Annual, III, Health Personnel and Hospital Establishments,* Geneva: WHO, 1975.

4

HEALTH MANPOWER: OTHER PERSONNEL

If the scope of this book permitted, it would be desirable to examine the numbers, training, and characteristics of all other types of health personnel in the same way we have considered the doctor. However, here we will consider only the highlights of the characteristics of some of the other major types of health worker. Because of their ancient origins and their persistent importance in most developing countries, the various types of traditional (i.e., nonscientific) healer will first be considered. Then we will summarize the main features of the nursing profession, which is the largest category of health worker trained formally throughout the world. Dental personnel of different levels and functions will be examined next. A variety of other secondary and auxiliary personnel—pharmacists, optometrists, midwives, and others—have evolved in most countries, and these must be described. Finally, one of the newest entrants into the health care field is what we may call the "doctor substitute," and this type of health worker, being trained increasingly in many countries, requires analysis.

Traditional Healers

While scientific medicine and its practice have evolved along the paths reviewed in previous chapters, traditional nonscientific healing has continued to be used throughout the world, remaining as a major source of medical care for the vast rural populations of the agricultural developing countries. To a lesser extent it is found also in the cities of those countries and even to some small extent among persons of limited education in all nations.

Anthropologists have given extensive accounts of the theoretical foundations and the practices of traditional healers in various primitive societies of all the continents. The treatments for disease and their rationales vary greatly among the *curanderos,* or healers, of various sections of Latin America, for example, of the Andean highland Indians, the jungle dwellers along the Amazon River in Brazil, and the *mestizo* communities of Mexico. All these, in turn, differ from the practices of voodoo practitioners or witch doctors of Africa or the *bomohs* of the Malay Peninsula (modern Malaysia). Much more systematized and having a recorded literature are the healing arts of the Ayurvedic and Unani practitioners of India and the traditional herbalists and acupuncturists of China.

In spite of these countless differences, one can distinguish certain main categories of traditional healers. There are those whose work is based on a theory of disease as a visitation from supernatural influences. Their treatments, therefore, invoke countervailing mystical powers through religious incantations or magic. The work of others is built on a theory of disease that may be partly empirical and partly philosophical. In Indian Ayurvedic healing, there are similarities to the pre-Hippocratic humors of Greek medicine, with treatment being designed to correct the imbalances that cause disease. Ancient Chinese medicine rests largely on the theory of interplay between the two great forces of *yang* (the male principle) and *ying* (the female principle), which are believed to operate throughout the universe as well as in the human body. It is the achievement of harmonious balance that is the object of therapy utilizing medications made from herbs or parts of animals.

Still other types of traditional healing are wholly empirical in foundation, being based on trial-and-error experience such as the ingestion of cinchona bark (quinine) for the treatment of malaria. The foxglove plant, containing digitalis, was a folk remedy for "dropsy" centuries before the action of digitalis, which reduced edema caused by heart failure, was understood. All sorts of treatments with heat and cold, with taking or avoiding certain foods, with rest or violent exercise, have had their origins in empirical observations.

Some traditional healing is a complex mixture of these magical, philosophical, and empirical principles. It is, furthermore, not static but influenced by the intrusion of modern scientific medicine. There are indigenous healers who have seen the "miracles" of penicillin for fevers and have added it to their repertoire without understanding microbiology. Some healers are, indeed, charlatans or quacks, who have no particular body of knowledge but who use whatever concoction they can formulate. Often it contains a fair dose of alcohol, making it not so different from Lydia E. Pinkham's Vegetable Compound (with 18 percent ethyl alcohol) on which millions of American women relied in the 1890s for their "monthly" troubles or for a wide range of "female ailments."

Whatever the type, traditional healers were for centuries the only resource for those seeking relief from sickness in the villages of the impoverished rural countries. As Western or scientific medicine has made its appearance, whether through a governmental health center, a religious missionary hospital, or an isolated trained doctor, the healer has not disappeared. He (less often than she) has been trusted by the people, whereas the "modern" doctor is strange. The village healer, moreover, is close at hand and inexpensive; he will take payment in the form of a chicken or a pot of grain or perhaps nothing at all. With many illnesses being self-limiting anyway, his ministrations may be followed by recovery even without any logic of cause-and-effect. The official, modern health center is likely to be not only far away, but it may be staffed by young doctors or nurses who seem alien and unsympathetic. Moreover, one may be kept waiting for hours on a hard bench before even being seen.

Anthropologists have described a typical sequence in the rural villager's reaction to sickness. First, he does nothing or takes the advice of a neighbor on diet or rest. If the symptoms persist, he visits a local healer or perhaps a second one in a neighboring village. Then, as a last resort, he makes the journey to a government health center where, more often than not, he will be tended by a young nursing auxiliary or other assistant health worker rather than a doctor. He takes medication dispensed in a bottle and, if he still continues to have symptoms, may start the cycle again. If he lives in or near a town where a pharmacy or a general food store with some drug stocks is located, this may be consulted also before or after he goes to the health center.

The working status of traditional healers varies. Some who have worked for many years and earned a good reputation are exclusively engaged in this activity. Others are farmers, small landowners, agricultural workers, or village merchants, who offer healing services as a part-time function. Although they are predominantly older men, some are women.

Closely related to the traditional healer is the village midwife, always a woman and usually the mother of several children of her own. She has learned her skills by observation and apprenticing to other midwives. Linked with her practices in delivering the baby are various traditional procedures designed to allay the pains of labor, to reduce bleeding, to assure a healthy baby, to hasten postpartum recovery, and so on. The infant's umbilical cord may be sealed off with a clean piece of cloth or with microbe-packed cow dung or mud. The mother's postpartum diet may be nutritious, or it may be devoid of needed protein for reasons of ancient custom.

Many developing countries, accepting reality, have attempted to train the traditional midwives in such elementary matters as maintaining sanitary conditions for delivering the mother and caring for the newborn baby, advising on a sound diet, detecting abnormalities of pregnancy that warrant referral to a hospital, and so on. At the same time, young women are being trained to carry out scientific midwifery, eventually to replace the traditional midwife.

Because of their anthropological interest and the light they shed on entire cultures, some anthropologists may have a tendency to exaggerate the importance of traditional healing in developing countries. As scientific health service has been extended, along with education of the people, the use of traditional healers has probably declined. As might be expected, older patients are more likely to resort to traditional healers, younger ones to scientific personnel. A nationwide household survey in Colombia in the 1960s found that of all contacts for medical help in the period of study (one month) only 17 percent of a random sample had consulted a traditional healer, in the rural areas, and only 4 percent in the cities. It is likely, however, that in India, Africa, or China, where the trained health manpower supply has been lower, these proportions would be higher.

Ideological remnants of traditional or nonscientific healing are found in virtually all societies to some degree. The American faith healer has been mentioned; there are also the chiropractor, the naturopath, or the food faddist. These healers presume to treat all ailments with single-track theories of disease that do not withstand scientific scrutiny. Yet, for reasons that combine mysticism with frustration with "regular" doctors, millions of people seek help from these cultist or sectarian practitioners. Other one-time cultists, such as osteopaths and homeopaths, have so modified their practices in the light of new knowledge that they use all the methods of scientific medicine, plus some techniques from their historical origins.

The responses of national health and scientific leaders to traditional healing differ. In Latin America and most of Africa, for example, the strategy has been to oppose them, to educate people against using them at all. In India, on the other hand, Ayurvedic medicine is so widespread and firmly entrenched that it is fully tolerated. In many Indian provinces, it is supported by government, with assistance given toward the maintenance of Ayurvedic training schools. Government laboratories test various Ayurvedic drugs, of which reserpine is probably the best known compound adopted widely by Western medicine. Little attempt, however, is made to integrate the ancient healing art with modern Indian medicine in day-to-day medical service.

In the People's Republic of China, since the revolutionary liberation of that huge country in 1949, another strategy has evolved. For the first fifteen years or so after liberation, a kind of neutral policy was followed, energies going mainly into building up scientific health manpower. Then around 1965, with progress in the vast rural areas (where 80 percent of the 750,000,000 people live) still unsatisfactory, Chairman Mao Tse-tung was quoted as referring to ancient Chinese medicine as a "great treasure house." It remained to be systematically explored, culling out the remedies of proven value and discarding the rest. In the meantime, Chairman Mao said, the policy should be to "combine traditional and Western medicine." This policy is implemented in many ways. Every Western-style medical school in China (eighty-five of them) contains a department of traditional medicine; similarly, the smaller number of traditional medicine schools each contains a department of Western medicine. In most modern hospitals and health centers, one or a few traditional doctors are also engaged, and the patient decides if he wishes to consult one of them.

Often Western and traditional doctors work in an outpatient clinic side-by-side, conferring with one another on the treatment of a case.

Skepticism long characterized the typical Western attitude toward traditional Chinese medicine, and Mao's dictum was regarded as a politically astute tactic for educating the traditional doctor about modern medical science. Then around 1968 the remarkable effectiveness of acupuncture anesthesia (or more accurately, analgesia) for major surgical operations burst upon the medical world. Although no one, least of all the Chinese, yet claims to know *how* it works, this unquestionable contribution of traditional Chinese healing to modern medical care is leading everyone to reserve judgment on the possible value of other ancient Chinese procedures or remedies. The staple of sympathetico-mimetic drugs, ephedrine, was an ancient Chinese contribution to modern pharmacology, and many more such contributions may lie ahead. More research clearly remains to be done.

Nurses

Religious sisters of the Catholic church, who took care of the sick and the destitute in the church-founded hospitals of the Middle Ages, were the precursors of modern nurses. Their goal was as much to show mercy to the suffering as an act of Christian charity on the pathway to the afterlife as to lessen the pain and discomfort of disease. The first formal training of women for nursing on a semireligious basis took place in Germany in 1836 and on a completely secular basis in London a little later. The work of Florence Nightingale in caring for soldiers in the Crimean War with a staff of trained young women is generally regarded as the origin of modern-day nursing. In 1860 she opened the first formal school of nursing at St. Thomas's Hospital in London.

As secular hospitals no longer under direct church control grew in Europe in the seventeenth and eighteenth centuries, the religious nuns had in large part been replaced by women of all sorts. Some of them were kindly ladies of upper class breeding who, with the *noblesse oblige* similar to that of the doctors, welcomed an opportunity to serve the poor; others were poor women who did the work for the benefit of the food and shelter they could gain for themselves. Neither group had technical training, and it was the concept of formal education pioneered by Florence Nightingale that opened a new era for this type of health personnel.

After 1860, schools of nursing spread rapidly through the hospitals of Europe, North America, then Australia and Japan. Unlike medicine, which was mainly university-based and used hospitals only for practical training, the education of nurses took place entirely in hospitals, instruction in technical subjects being given by the doctors and in the personal aspects of patient care by the more seasoned nurses. To upgrade the entire quality of the field, the prerequisite for entry to a nursing school came to be completion of secondary school education. The first nursing school making this requirement in the United States was started at the municipal Bellevue Hospital, New York City, in 1873.

As hospitals expanded in the late nineteenth and early twentieth centuries, nursing schools were established in almost all the larger ones, if only to provide a steady flow of trained young women to staff each hospital. It soon became apparent that training as a nurse was also an excellent preparation for marriage, not only because it provided the young woman with numerous skills but because it brought her into contact with young men—doctors, patients, and others—in search of wives. As a result, the professional life of a graduate nurse became quite short, only three or four years, before she left the nursing field for marriage responsibilities, and new waves of nurses had to be continuously trained. With hospitals ever expanding, the treadmill of nursing education had to move faster and faster to keep up with the needs.

It was in 1916 that Great Britain first created a governmental Registry of Nurses (hence, the RN), but it soon became apparent that the enlarging needs of hospitals for such fully trained nurses could no longer be met. Public health agencies, visiting nurse associations, and even private doctors in their offices were making further demands. By around 1920, therefore, hospitals began training other women, with lesser prior education, in shorter curricula (often one year instead of the three years that had become conventional) for nursing duties. These were called "practical nurses," rather than "registered," and they became widely used as auxiliaries to the registered nurse. Eventually several governments established official certification for them also, as "licensed practical nurses" (LPNs) or licensed vocational nurses (LVNs). New York State first formalized such licensure in America in 1938.

Even this adjustment did not solve the hospital personnel needs, and a third class of nurse's aide arose. She was typically a woman with no formal training, except a sort of on-the-job apprenticeship to a registered nurse. Thus, in many industrialized countries there developed three classes of hospital-trained nurses: the registered nurse, the practical or vocational nurse, and the nurse's aide.

After World War II, a fourth class of nurse emerged in the United States, the university graduate nurse with a bachelor's degree. She (occasionally, he) is trained for leadership positions in education, administration, and public health functions, but this pattern was emulated in only a few other affluent nations. A handful of baccalaureate nurses had actually been trained at the University of Minnesota in 1909, but the idea did not take hold until forty years later.

After World War II, another change occurred in nursing education, originating in the United States and then spreading to other economically

advanced nations, especially in the British Commonwealth. This was the shift
of the locale of training the RN from the three-year hospital school to the two-
year junior college. Starting slowly in a few states, such as California and New
York where junior colleges were numerous, the movement gradually gained
momentum. It was believed that in the academic setting of a junior or community college the student nurse could learn more in two years than in three
years spent in the work-oriented and less didactic setting of the busy hospital.
Besides, hospital schools of nursing were getting very expensive to operate.
Hence, by 1962 about 4 percent of registered nurses graduated in the United
States came from junior colleges, and by 1973 this figure had shot up to 42
percent.

This alteration in nursing education did not characterize the developing
countries or the socialist countries. In Africa, in India, the Middle East, and
Latin America, there is not the pattern of the junior or community college.
After secondary school (often termed in French or Spanish-speaking countries
"college"), the student goes to a full-fledged university. Here medicine might
be studied or law or engineering or economics but not nursing. In these developing countries, the education of nurses has remained a hospital function. One
influence of the industrialized countries (mediated to some extent through the
World Health Organization) that might be seriously questioned is the prerequisite of secondary schooling for the training of the registered or "professional
nurse" in a three-year hospital course. As a result, very few applicants come
along. The relatively rare young woman who completes secondary school in a
developing country and seeks further education wants to go on to higher-status
university training; nursing is looked upon in these countries as a rather lowly
calling, especially in middle-class families.

As a result, in the developing countries of Latin America or Asia or Africa,
registered nurses are scarce. Whereas in the United States or Europe, there are
two or three registered nurses to each doctor, in most other countries there are
conversely two or three doctors to each registered nurse. Nursing service, in
other words, must be given predominantly by young women with very little
training—typically elementary school (four to six years) followed by a few
months of special training. These young women are considered auxiliary nurses
or nursing assistants, and they are usually prepared in hospitals or at other special training centers operated by ministries of health. The hospital-trained registered nurses in these countries are so scarce that they are usually reserved for
supervisory positions in large hospitals or in public health agencies.

The urban-rural disparity of registered nurses is also extreme in the developing countries. Since the RN with secondary schooling is usually from an urban
background, she tends to work in a city hospital at the elbow of the doctor.
Meanwhile, the nursing assistants needed to staff the small rural hospitals, health
centers, or rural health posts are drawn from the villages; their supervision from

a doctor is episodic. Yet these young women, with much more cursory training, are expected to carry heavy independent responsibility, often including primary medical care. It is an inequity that is tolerated only because of different health care standards being applied to different social classes.

Canada and Norway are among the few countries training a special type of nurse for psychiatric service. She or he receives the same length of training, following secondary school graduation, as a registered nurse, but the training takes place in a mental hospital. The certification is as a psychiatric nurse or PN, and such nurses carry a major part of the patient-care load in mental hospitals. In addition to learning about the general care of sick patients, these nurses are trained in the special problems of the mentally ill.

Dental Personnel

There is a serious shortage of dental personnel throughout the world. Even in the wealthiest of nations, the United States, there are not enough dentists to meet the basic needs, which explains why even health insurance programs so seldom provide for access to dental care. A high proportion of American children do not see a dentist once a year, even though the United States has one of the highest number of dentists—about 1 to 2,000 people—of any nation. Norway has most dentists, with a ratio of 1:1,200. In the countries of Africa, the dentist-population ratio is about 1:65,000; in Asia it is about 1:17,000. Even in Europe as a whole it is only 1:3,500.

The most practical and effective approach to the dentist shortage has been pioneered by New Zealand. In 1920 this small country in the South Pacific started a program of training dental nurses to work in the schools and give complete dental care to children. Following high school, the dental nurse receives two years of training in a special center. Her functions are far broader than those performed by the dental hygienist (first trained in America in 1916 and found now in Europe and elsewhere) whose work is largely confined to cleaning teeth. The dental nurse does fillings, extractions (rarely necessary), and of course prophylactic work under the only occasional supervision of a dentist. By being located with her equipment in the schools, she is able to serve large numbers of children routinely with a minimum loss of time. The quality of her work has been found to be highly satisfactory by impartial observers from the World Health Organization, even though it is done more slowly than that done by a dentist. In some countries, this form of dental worker is known as a dental therapist or dental auxiliary, but her functions are still far broader than those of the hygienist or chairside dental assistant.

Although the dental nurse idea has been highly controversial in many countries, it has been emulated enthusiastically in about twenty other nations, mainly those in the British Commonwealth, most recently in several provinces of Canada. The two-year training program of the dental nurse is, of course, far less costly than the five- to eight-year university training required for a professional dentist, and her work is remunerated at a much more modest level than that of the dentist, whether he is paid by fees or salary. Even if the professional life of a dental nurse is only five to ten years, much shorter than a dentist's, the cost-benefit ratio is better. Moreover, it has simply not been found possible to attract enough of the available supply of dentists into the field of working with children.

Although the ratio of dentists to population has not increased at the same rate as that of physicians, and in some countries (including the United States) it has even declined in recent years, the net output of dental service has increased. The reason is a much expanded use of chairside dental assistants and the availability of more efficient equipment, such as high-speed drills. Dental assistants were for many years trained on the job in dental offices or clinics, but since about 1920 special courses of one or two years have been offered. There are twenty-three such dental assistant training programs in the United States, where this service is most highly developed.

The dental technician or dental mechanic is the person who prepares dental prostheses—partial or complete dentures to replace the natural teeth. In the economically advanced countries, these personnel (usually men) work in dental laboratories on the basis of castings submitted by dentists. In the poorer countries, however, and even to some extent in poor districts of developed countries (e.g., Australia and Canada), one finds "denturists," persons who provide complete upper and/or lower dentures to patients whose teeth have been totally extracted. Essentially, denturists are dental mechanics to whom the population has direct access at much lower costs than through the channel of a dentist. Although not officially licensed to do this work, the denturist is a social response to the need for complete dentures (false teeth) by poor people.

In the Soviet Union and some other socialist countries, there are two levels of what Americans would call dentist. There is the stomatologist, who is essentially a medical faculty graduate, specializing in disorders of the mouth. In 1963, the USSR had 20,300 of these. Second is the dental doctor, who is trained in a secondary type of technical school for a shorter period. There were 37,300 of these in 1963. In general, the simpler work of fillings, extractions, cleanings, and the like is done by the dental doctor, whereas the more complex rehabilitative oral work, as well as more difficult diagnostic problems, are handled by the stomatologist. In large centers, several dental doctors may work under the general supervision of a stomatologist, but most dental doctors work in health centers or polyclinics, without special supervision, and refer complicated cases to a stomatologist.

Despite the clear evidence of the benefits of fluoridated water in prevention of dental caries, most countries have not yet implemented this simple and

effective preventive health measure. More surprising, perhaps, is the objection
by professional dentists in most countries, including the United States, to the
development of the dental nurse or therapist, even though her work is confined
to children and has been found to be highly effective. In all the approximately
twenty countries where this type of dental worker has been trained, she functions in an organized framework, on salary and under some supervision, rather
than as an independent practitioner. Yet there seems to be fear that she will
constitute a low-priced form of competition to the dentist, although the objections articulated by dentists usually focus on the quality of her work. It is difficult to understand this reasoning when we know that under present arrangements, the majority of children in even the wealthy countries and the overwhelming mass of children in the poor countries grow to adulthood with grossly
inadequate or totally lacking dental care.

Other Secondary and Auxiliary Personnel

The types and numbers of other secondary and auxiliary personnel for health
service, beyond those already discussed, are too great to discuss in detail. These
personnel are characterized by specialized functions in relation to certain parts
of the body or certain technologies, whether or not they are auxiliary to the
doctor or directly accessible to the patient.

As noted in the preceding chapter, visual refractions in many countries
have become the special province of personnel called optometrists, opticians,
or sometimes dispensing opticians or optical dispensers. Ordinarily, the patient
may go directly to these practitioners without a doctor's referral, but the scope
of work they are permitted to do (e.g., use of eye drops or measurement of intra-
ocular pressure) varies among countries. In general, the influence of physicians,
particularly ophthalmologists (sometimes called oculists), has been to call for
legislation restricting their functions as much as possible, while the optometrists
have fought for widening their role. In the British scene, where both these
types of personnel work together as a team, this controversy is not found.

As populations become more educated and interested in reading, the
demand for visual refractions increases. In virtually all countries, there is a need
for more optometrists. There is hardly a clearer example of wastage of medical
manpower than the large allocation of time for refractive work by medical ophthalmologists. Yet, the pattern of private fee-for-service medical practice per-
petuates this extravagance.

The podiatrist or chiropodist is rarely found outside the highly developed
countries or the metropolitan centers of other countries. In a sense, he is a
health worker in response to the "civilized" practice of wearing shows. Most
disorders of the feet come from unhygienic frictions and pressures from ill-fitting

footwear; a whole industry has arisen in the most affluent nations to provide patients with individually moulded shoes in order to correct the disorders arising from ordinary shoes. In countries without podiatrists, surgical correction of bunions or other disorders of the feet, especially in aged patients, is done by doctors. The major difference among the relatively few countries with podiatrists and chiropodists is in their period of training: in Great Britain, for example (where they are typically called chiropodists), the training period is two years in a technical school. In the United States, with its general tendency to upgrade all health occupations, the usual training required is two years of college followed by a four-year university course leading to a doctorate of podiatric medicine (DPM) degree. The same upward movement of the health disciplines is seen in nursing, speech therapy, and other disciplines in the affluent, free-market-dominated American economy.

The midwife, both the traditional and the trained types, is far more commonly used throughout the world than one would gather from the American scene. The custom in the United States, for both indigenous and trained midwives, has been for them to perform deliveries in the mother's home. In Europe and many formerly colonial countries, however, although traditional midwives do deliveries solely in the home, trained midwives render service both in the home and the hospital. In British hospitals, for example, the vast majority of normal deliveries (except primiparae), as well as the prenatal care, are done by midwives. Obstetricians confine their work mainly to abnormal pregnancies and to primiparae. The same is true in Holland, Norway, and some regions of France. In Malaysia, Indonesia, India, and most of Africa this is also the practice.

In the rural villages of the developing countries, the majority of all childbirths are still attended in the home by traditional midwives. Even when trained government midwives are stationed in the villages at small, attractive health stations, it tends to be a long time before pregnant women turn to them for help, in place of the traditional midwives used by their mothers. To adjust to these realities, many developing countries offer short courses of training for traditional midwives to teach them the elements of hygiene in the delivery process and care of the newborn. This strategy has been successful in reducing infant and maternal mortality.

The pharmacist, descendant of the ancient apothecary, is probably the oldest health worker besides the doctor. As recently as the early nineteenth century, most low-income people in Europe, the majority of the population, would typically first consult an apothecary for their ailments, not only because he was less expensive than the physician, but also because he was considered the greater expert on drugs. A great lore of secrecy, guarded zealously by apothecaries and even doctors, was associated with sickness remedies. Sometimes affluent patients would go directly to an apothecary for what they considered minor ailments.

In Europe and later in North America, it was the late nineteenth century before the custom and eventually legal statutes developed that required medical prescriptions to authorize the pharmacist to dispense certain drugs. As we know to this day, many common drugs are dispensed over the counter without prescriptions. And in the developing countries, where drug control legislation is typically lax or even nonexistent, almost any drug (except perhaps narcotics) can be obtained by the patient directly from a pharmacist, often a store-keeper without any pharmaceutical training, without a physician's order. On the other hand, in rural regions of even the wealthy nations, where pharmacies are scarce or lacking, the private doctor or the health center will dispense its own drugs as an integral part of the medical service. In Japan, even in the main cities, drug dispensing is typically done by the private doctor; the Japanese health insurance programs encourage this by their system of fee payments. To multiply patient visits, since the fee per visit is rather low, Japanese doctors typically dispense small quantities of drugs even for minor ailments, thus requiring the patient to return soon for an additional supply.

With the pharmaceutical industry expanding rapidly, especially in the United States and Europe, and with more sophisticated preparation and packaging of various drug compounds and mixtures, the role of the pharmacist has inevitably changed in the last fifty to seventy-five years. The symbolic mortar and pestle, with which the nineteenth century pharmacist prepared his compounds of multiple ingredients, are rarely used because prepackaged pills and compounds are produced in countless variety by the pharmaceutical manufacturer. Automated production in large factories is far more efficient, and probably more accurate, so that the need for local pharmacists has actually declined— the striking exception to the rule of expanding demands for health personnel. This helps to explain the common combination of drug dispensing with the sale of cosmetics, candy, and all sorts of drugstore sundries, although this is less frequent in Europe. It also helps to explain the search of the modern pharmacist in the economically advanced countries for a new identity.

With his role as drug dispenser so reduced, the serious pharmacist is in search of new professional functions. One path has been development of the role of clinical pharmacist, that is, the expert in the enormous multiplicity of new drugs and the hazards of their harmful interactions. This role is performed more easily in hospitals, where all of a patient's medications are conveniently listed on one chart, but it is more difficult in the community, where a patient may see several doctors and go to several different pharmacies. If patients were to use only one pharmacy (regardless of the number of doctors consulted) and a tabulation were kept on each patient's medications, the pharmacist could be on the alert to detect possible drug interactions that might be unknown to the diverse prescribing doctors. The pharmacist could then inform the several doctors and advise on drug choices that would avoid negative effects.

Another new role for the pharmacist sought by some leaders is to train him and encourage his role as a community health educator. The pharmacist is naturally in an excellent position to educate people about health problems—both those for which they come to his premises for help and others. He can also explain to the patient the best manner to take prescribed drugs, something often overlooked by the busy doctor. In developing countries, it is common for pharmacists for a small fee to give injections even of drugs not medically prescribed. They also perform simple diagnostic tests, such as urinalyses or blood pressure determinations, sometimes even as part of organized case-detection campaigns. In Australia, pharmacists play the unusual role of collecting premiums for official health insurance funds. All in all, the pharmacist's role is in flux, for the pharmaceutical industry has largely eliminated his traditional functions.

The vast majority of the world's drugs are manufactured, or their basic chemicals are produced, in North America and Europe. As a result, the developing countries, composing most of the world's population, have become heavily dependent on importation of drugs, which tend to be costly. Whereas drugs may typically constitute 10 to 15 percent of health care expenditures in the United States or Europe, they may consume 33 percent or more of health costs in Latin America or Africa. Even the American or European firms located on the outskirts of Guatemala City or Accra are simply for packaging the pharmaceutical chemicals imported from abroad but still sold locally at relatively high prices. Only in a few poor countries, such as India or the People's Republic of China, have the complex tasks of complete domestic fabrication of antibiotics, contraceptive pills, and other important medications been achieved.

Still other types of allied health worker are the various forms of support personnel for diagnostic and treatment services. These include laboratory and x-ray technicians and persons skilled in electrocardiography (ECG) or electro-encephalography (EEG). They include the various rehabilitation workers for physical, occupational, and speech therapy. They include social workers, medical and psychiatric. They include inhalation therapists, plaster cast technicians, audiologists, remedial gymnasts, and other such highly specialized technicians. They include psychologists, nutritionists, medical record librarians, and brace-makers. All these and other special workers in selected aspects of comprehensive modern medicine are most abundant by far in the highly developed countries. In the poorer countries, these roles are often played by more generalized health workers, especially nurses or the general variety of medical assistant or doctor substitute previously mentioned and discussed below in more detail.

Perhaps the most recently recognized category of support personnel in the health services throughout the world is the specialist in health service administration. For centuries it was assumed that the top administrative authority in any organized health program, either within institutional walls or on a community basis, had to be a physician. He might be assisted by fiscal or other administrative aides, but final authority rested with the doctor. This policy still prevails in many countries, especially the poorer ones where the market for private medical services has not been so great. It was in the United States that the first formal training programs developed for public health administrators, and later hospital administrators, who were not necessarily physicians.

When the first American school of public health was pioneered (jointly between Harvard and the Massachusetts Institute of Technology) in 1916 and the first school of hospital administration was established at the University of Chicago in 1934, the focus was primarily to train physicians for administrative responsibilities. Gradually, as the demands for effective administrators increased more rapidly than the supply of physicians who chose to enter this work (in the face of the generally much more lucrative rewards of private practice), persons with other academic backgrounds were welcomed into these schools. In the schools of public health, it was first other health professionals such as dentists, nurses, or veterinarians, then pharmacists or laboratory technologists, and now a wide spectrum of persons from social science backgrounds. In the programs of hospital administration (some located within schools of public health but most under the auspices of schools of business administration or other academic entities), applicants were welcome from backgrounds in accounting, business management, or other such fields. For many years, physicians from Latin America and all the developing continents were sent to American universities for such public health or hospital administration training. Gradually, especially since World War II, schools for such training of health administrators—as well as other community-oriented specialists in epidemiology, sanitation, nutrition, statistics, and the like—have been established on every continent.

Finally, in the sphere of community health work there is a wide spectrum of specialized but rather briefly trained personnel for very restricted functions. There are sanitarians or sanitary inspectors for environmental control work. In the United States they are often trained to the bachelor's degree level, but in most countries they get a brief year or so of instruction after secondary school or even primary school. To control malaria, the minimally trained DDT house-sprayer is widely used in developing tropical countries. The vaccinator is trained for the single task of smallpox inoculation. In population control programs the family-planning adviser is trained. Depending on the epidemiological circumstances, other workers with restricted tasks are trained for the attack on particular insects or other disease vectors or even for dispensing special medications.

Doctor Substitutes

For much broader functions, especially in the poor and predominantly rural countries, another type of health worker has been trained to meet a wide range of needs. To emphasize this role, rather than the restricted functions of the personnel discussed above, we have chosen to call this health worker a doctor substitute. He or she performs mainly for rural populations, the same or almost the same scope of functions ordinarily expected of the general medical practitioner. Rather than being truly auxiliary to the doctor for certain techniques or the management of certain conditions, the doctor substitute works largely independently as the primary health worker, through whom the rural patient enters the total health service system. This type of health worker is also not to be confused with the traditional healer who likewise aims to treat all disease but who receives no scientific training and is, in any case, not part of the general health care system.

It was in Czarist Russia in the 1860s that the idea of doctor substitutes was first developed. To serve the large rural population of that country, after the abolition of serfdom in 1867, a system of rural *zemstvo* or district medical care was established at government expense. Each district was headed by a salaried doctor, but under his direction were several field assistants or *feldshers,* stationed in villages around the district. The *feldshers* were drawn from medical corpsmen who had completed their military duty in the Czarist armies (similar to the physician assistants of the 1960s drawn from American veterans of the Vietnam War). The *feldsher's* training had been received mainly in the army, but he received a little further training from the *zemstvo* doctor.

Despite the *feldsher's* limited training, the prevailing philosophy of Czarist Russia was that the *feldsher* was good enough for the peasants, whose ailments were considered simpler than those of city dwellers. Besides, *feldshers* were much less expensive for the government to support than physicians, even if the latter could be persuaded to work in rural areas. When the Soviet system of socialized health services was developed after the 1917 revolution, it was initially decided to eliminate the *feldsher* as constituting second-class medicine. But the problems of training enough doctors to serve the rural population were so great that, in the end, the policy implemented was to retain the *feldsher,* give him much more systematic training, and back him up with reliable medical supervision. There have been various ups and downs in the attitudes toward and the training of Soviet *feldshers* over the years, and in the rural areas his or her role (today many women are trained) tends to be broader than in the cities, but over 400,000 *feldshers* currently work in a variety of doctor replacement roles in the Soviet health system. However, it is noteworthy that in recent years, as the number of doctors has increased, the USSR and other socialist countries have phased out the training of new *feldshers.* The existing ones are being directed into such specialized functions as technicians, ambulance attendants, or sanitarians.

In the European colonies of Africa, for reasons similar to those of the

Russian Czarist regime, the elementary doctor substitute was used extensively. In the nineteenth century, the only fully trained physicians were the white men from the ruling country, and they served mainly in the principal cities. (Exceptions were the medical missionaries who, like Albert Schweitzer from Belgium, set up their hospitals in the hinterland.) When rural health posts were established by the colonial medical systems, they were staffed by male medical assistants or dressers, who had learned some surgical techniques assisting the white doctors in hospitals—hence, dressers—and in the same way learned about the commonly used drugs. Their training, however, was seldom formalized.

After independence was gained by most of the African countries following World War II, the organizational principles of the former British, French, Belgian, or other colonial medical systems were largely carried over. A major policy change, however, was to provide more systematic training to the dressers or the various medical assistants designated by other names, such as *officiers de santé* (health officers). These personnel, typically young African men, are now taught to emphasize preventive services, giving immunizations, advice on environmental sanitation, and some health education. They have learned to provide certain basic drugs for fevers, diarrheas, respiratory disorders, and so on, even if their guidelines to treatment are mainly symptoms rather than etiologic diagnoses. There are so few physicians in Africa that, in practice, these health workers get very little supervision; if a patient's sickness persists he is sent, if transportation is available, to a hospital, which is usually distant.

The Latin American nursing auxiliary, mentioned earlier, although theoretically a doctor's helper in patient care (like other nurses), in practice often serves as an elementary doctor substitute in rural villages. Although such doctor substitutes are usually young village women, in some Latin American countries men trained originally as sanitary inspectors may be given a bit of clinical orientation and sent out to staff rural health posts in the same way. A more recent personnel development in several Latin American countries is the *promotore de salud* or health promoter. Pioneered in Venezuela under the slogan of *medicina simplificada* (simplified medicine), this health worker is deliberately trained for clinical duties, without the pretense of serving as a nurse. Elementary school (six grades) completion is usually required, and the training program lasts about six months. U.S. Peace Corps nurses and doctors have also trained such rural health promoters in some countries, such as Ecuador. In Guatemala a more elaborate program for training *técnicos de salud rural* (rural health technicians or TSR's) has recently been launched, requiring completion of secondary school and two years of training.

In Ethiopia, since about 1955, there has been a program for training primary health workers or doctor substitutes to a much higher level than the dresser of colonial heritage. It is significant perhaps that, except for a brief period under Italian domination, Ethiopia did not have a colonial tradition.

Located at the mountain town of Gondar, the Haile Selassie Public Health College and Training Center gives a three-year course to young men who have completed secondary school (twelve grades). Graduates are then appointed as health
officers in charge of rural health centers. Their responsibilities combine preventive, treatment, and administrative functions. Trained auxiliary nurses and sanitarians are also in the health centers. With very few doctors available, these
personnel inevitably make fewer referrals than, for example, the Soviet *feldsher*
or the Latin American health promoter. Meanwhile, it is interesting to note that
Ethiopia, like other African nations, continues to train and use some dressers—
young men with one year of hospital training after six years of elementary
school. A center somewhat like the Gondar college was developed in British
Fiji some years ago for training native doctors, but it was later converted to a
full-fledged medical school.

It appears that, through an evolutionary process, former British colonies,
now British Commonwealth nations, have come to develop more advanced
training programs for doctor substitutes. (This is aside from their formation
of medical schools in the national capitals.) In Ceylon, for example, the original medical assistant, called an apothecary because of his role as drug dispenser in a hospital, was gradually upgraded with a course of two years following
secondary school (eleven grades). Today these men are assigned to rural health
posts, with wide preventive, diagnostic, and curative responsibilities, and designated as assistant medical practitioners. Similarly, in Malaysia, another former
British colony, the mainstay for primary medical care in the rural areas is the
hospital assistant. His training, originally by apprenticeship, is now equivalent
in length to that of the graduate nurse (three years after secondary school) but
different in content. He is taught to diagnose and treat disease with drugs and
to do minor surgery but not preventive work. The latter is done by nurses or
nursing assistants who work along with him in rural health centers. Fully
trained physicians are theoretically responsible for the operation of sets of five
health centers, but they visit each only once a week at the most. Difficult cases
are asked to return to see the doctor at his next scheduled visit.

It should be apparent that in these developing countries there is a manifest
delineation of health care responsibilities among allied health workers along sex
lines. Personal preventive services, especially for babies and expectant mothers,
are mainly given by women, as various levels of nurse, but the diagnosis and
treatment of disease in any patient are usually performed by men. One can
hardly doubt that this policy springs from the prejudices of male-dominated
societies, in which women are not entrusted with the more critical decisions,
such as treating the sick. It is also related to the historic origins of many of the
doctor substitutes in the military services—such as the original nineteenth century
Russian *feldsher*, the African dresser, or the latterday American Medex from the
Vietnam War. (It is noteworthy that in America the nurse-practitioner with

broad clinical functions did not arise until the physician's assistant had first broken the ice on the doctor substitute concept.)

When emancipation or liberation of women has become a top national priority, as it did in the postrevolutionary Soviet Union or in modern Cuba, this policy abruptly changes. Not only are half or over half the Soviet *feldshers* women, but more than 50 percent of the new graduate doctors in the Soviet Union and Cuba are likewise women. The same applies in the People's Republic of China, where thousands of middle medical personnel on the *feldsher* model were trained soon after the 1949 Revolution.

Since 1965 there has been developed a highly innovative form of doctor substitute who is having enormous impact on world-wide thinking about rural health services. In 1965, only some sixteen years after its revolution, brewings emerged in China about a rise of bureaucracy and elitism in the government that led to the Proletarian Cultural Revolution of 1966-1970. As part of this major shakeup in Chinese Communist leadership, there was a basic reappraisal of rural health services that were still found to be substantially poorer than urban services. To correct this, rural districts around Shanghai conceived the idea of a massive program of short training—three to six months—of selected peasants to perform basic and elementary curative and preventive health services. Each such health worker was to continue his or her work in the fields and render health services only part of the time to about 400 to 600 persons in a production brigade (a component of an agricultural commune). The idea quickly spread and, under the label of barefoot doctor, a nationwide policy emerged. Candidates for this training are chosen by the members of the production brigade and need no prerequisites except literacy. The training is given in the nearest district hospital or health center, and each year a refresher course of one to two weeks is taken. Physicians from the city hospitals move out to the communes for periods of one to two years to carry out this training, and at any one time about one-third of hospital doctors are away doing this work. The barefoot doctors are paid not by the central or provincial governments but by their own communes, in the same way as they are paid for their agricultural work. In the factories, somewhat equivalent worker doctors have been trained, and elsewhere in the cities are red medical workers (usually housewives).

The barefoot doctor idea, emphasizing rapidly acquired and practical skills rather than theoretical knowledge, has seized the imagination of health leaders throughout the developing world. More than a million such persons, it is claimed, have already been trained in People's China, a ratio of about 1:500 rural people. In addition to immunizations, family planning, and other preventive services, the barefoot doctor treats common ailments with both Western drugs and traditional herbal remedies, as well as using acupuncture occasionally. Perplexing cases are referred to a health center or hospital staffed by full-fledged physicians. Furthermore, if his or her work is well regarded, the barefoot doctor may be recommended by the commune for admission to a regular medical school. The program has been heralded by the World Health Organization and encouraged for development in other predominantly rural countries.

This completes a general overview of health manpower throughout the world. It is evident that the types, numbers, and functions of doctors and allied health personnel differ with the patterns for health service financing and delivery in each country. These patterns are, in turn, determined by each nation's socioeconomic level and political system. Improvements in the provision of health manpower to meet population needs obviously depend on an understnading of these dynamics.

Readings

Badgley, Robin F. et al., "International Studies of Health Manpower: A Sociologic Perspective," *Medical Care, 9*:235-252 (May-June 1971).

Baker, Timothy D. and Mark Perlman, *Health Manpower in a Developing Economy: Taiwan, A Case Study in Planning,* Baltimore: Johns Hopkins Press, 1967.

Bennett, F. J. et al., "Manpower in East Africa—Prospects and Problems," *East African Medical Journal, 42*:149-161 (April 1965).

Bullough, Bonnie and Vern Bullough, *Issues in Nursing,* New York: Springer Co., 1966.

Bullough, Vern L. and Bonnie Bullough, *The Emergence of Modern Nursing,* New York: Macmillan Co., 1969.

Chang, Wen-Pin, "Health Manpower Development in an African Country: The Case of Ethiopia," *Journal of Medical Education, 45*:29-39 (January 1970).

Cohen, Lois K. and E. Barmes, "International Collaborative Study of Dental Manpower Systems in Relation to Oral Health Status," *Social Science and Medicine, 8*:325-327 (May 1974).

Fendall, N. R. E., "The Medical Assistant in Africa," *Journal of Tropical Medicine & Hygiene, 71*:83-95 (April 1968).

——, *Auxiliaries in Health Care: Programs in Developing Countries,* Baltimore: Johns Hopkins Press, 1972.

Gish, Oscar, *Health Manpower and the Medical Auxiliary,* London: Intermediate Technology Development Group, 1971.

——, "Doctor Auxiliaries in Tanzania," *The Lancet,* 1 December 1973, pp. 1251-1254.

Hall, Thomas L., *Health Manpower in Peru—New Approaches to an Old Problem,* Baltimore: Johns Hopkins Press, 1969.

——, "Chile Health Manpower Study: Methods and Problems," *International Journal of Health Services, 1*'362-377 (1971).

Huard, P., "Western Medicine and Afro-Asian Ethnic Medicine" in *Medicine and Culture,* F. N. L. Poynter (ed.), London: Wellcome Institute, 1965.

King, Maurice (ed.), *Medical Care in Developing Countries,* Nairobi: Oxford University Press, 1966.

Kremers, E. and G. Urdung, *History of Pharmacy,* Philadelphia, 1940.

Long, E. C. and Alberto Viau, "Health Care Extension Using Medical Auxiliaries in Guatemala," *The Lancet,* 26 January 1974, pp. 127-130.

McGilvray, J. C., "Health Services and Health Manpower for the Developing Countries," *World Hospitals, 6*:1-4 (1970).

Organization for Economic Cooperation & Development, *Study of Education of the Professions in the Context of Health Care Systems,* Paris: OECD, October 1974.

Pan American Health Organization, *Medical Auxiliaries,* Washington, D.C.: PAHO, Scientific Pub. No. 278, 1973.

Pene, P., "Health Auxiliaries in Francophone Africa," *The Lancet,* 12 May 1973, pp. 1047-1048.

Roemer, Milton I., "The Role of Allied Health Manpower in Developing and Socialist Countries," *Journal of Allied Health, 3*:77-85 (Summer 1974).

Roemer, Milton and Ruth Roemer, *Health Manpower under National Health Insurance: The Canadian Experience,* Washington, D.C.: U.S. Health Resources Administration, 1976.

Roemer, Ruth and Milton I. Roemer, *Health Manpower in the Changing Australian Health Services Scene,* Washington, D.C.: U.S. Health Resources Administration, 1975.

Ronaghy, H. A., "Is the Chinese 'Barefoot Doctor' Exportable to Rural Iran?" *The Lancet,* 29 June 1974, pp. 1331-1333.

Sidel, Victor W., "Feldshers and Feldsherism: The Role and Training of the Feldsher in the U.S.S.R.," *New England Journal of Medicine, 278*:934-940, 981-992 (1968).

———, "The Barefoot Doctors of the People's Republic of China," *New England Journal of Medicine, 286*:1292-1300 (1972).

Sundram, C. J., "The Delivery of Dental Services in the Asian Area of the Pacific Basin," *International Dental Journal, 23*:555-558 (December 1973).

Taylor, Carl E., R. Dirican, and K. W. Deuschle, *Health Manpower Planning in Turkey,* Baltimore: Johns Hopkins Press, 1968.

Vaughn, J. P., "Are Doctors Always Necessary? A Review of the Need for the Medical Assistant in Developing Countries," *Journal of Tropical Medicine and Hygiene, 74*:265-271 (December 1971).

Walser, H. H. and H. M. Koelbing (eds.), *Erwin Ackerknecht: Medicine and Ethnology,* Bern: Huber, 1971.

World Health Organization, *The Development of Studies in Health Manpower* (Report of a WHO Scientific Group), Geneva: WHO Tech. Report Series No. 481, 1971.

5

HEALTH FACILITIES

In all countries health facilities have been developed to provide a framework in which doctors and other health personnel can do their work effectively. Most important are hospitals, to bring together manpower and equipment for care of the seriously sick, but hospitals are being increasingly used for further health purposes as well. Because they mobilize resources this way, hospitals and other health facilities invariably become more than merely buildings but also organized centers of authority and responsibility for health services.

Since health professionals do so much of their work in hospitals, it is important that they understand how these complex organizations operate. To convey this understanding, this chapter will consider briefly the historical background of hospitals throughout the world. This background accouts for variable mixtures of hospital sponsorship and ownership in different countries, which will be examined. Then we will discuss the various types of hospital and the functions of each type. The methods of administration and financing of hospital services in different national settings will also be considered. Regionalization is an important concept by which hospitals are systematically planned in most countries, and this will be discussed. Finally we will consider briefly health centers for the organized provision of ambulatory care, and other special types of health facility, such as pharmacies and laboratories.

History of Hospitals

The historical development of hospitals reflects the evolution of medical science and also the changing attitudes of society toward disease. These attitudes have often differed with respect to various population groups and are reflected in the special types of hospital that have been developed. In ancient Greece there were semireligious temples of healing that were devoted to Aesculapius (or in Greek,

Asklepios), the god of medicine. The sick would come with offerings to pray and rest. Later in the Roman Empire, there were hospitals for wounded or sick soldiers and also *valetudinaria* (field shelters) for slaves, whose recovery from sickness meant a preservation of productive manpower. However, hospitals of today are usually traced to medieval Europe, where the Christian church established hostels to shelter the sick, the aged, and the poor. Some hostels were associated with monasteries, others with cathedrals in the main cities. A somewhat similar development, inspired by religious motives but less directly linked to the religious organization, developed in the Moslem world. As hospitals grew in the cities and as urban populations increased, the cost of operating these facilities naturally rose. Therefore, even though their ownership and control remained religious, financial support was given by local governments. As early as the sixteenth century, representatives of local authorities were appointed to hospital boards of directors.

Later city governments began to establish hospitals themselves. With medical science developing in the seventeenth and eighteenth centuries, hospitals expanded under both religious and secular authorities, the latter acquiring increasing importance. In Latin America, which was colonized mainly by Spain and Portugal (where the Catholic church was very strong), religious sponsorship was carried over, numerous charitable or *beneficencia* hospitals being founded. In the British and French colonies of Asia and Africa, the hospitals under colonial authorities were mainly governmental.

In the early nineteenth century, a new type of hospital sponsorship emerged: the voluntary nonsectarian institution. A group of citizens, often led by one or two large benefactors, would establish a general hospital without the involvement of either church or state. Financial support came from charitable donations and later by government subsidy. With non-indigent patients beginning to use hospitals, private fees were also being collected. This pattern became prominent in England and in British colonies overseas, including North America, Australia, and India.

In the late nineteenth and early twentieth centuries, the rise of social insurance began to influence hospitals. This source of relatively stable economic support for medical care of workers and often their dependents led to the financial strengthening of hospitals in some countries. Polyclinics for specialized medicine were constructed directly by social insurance groups, and later these clinics added their own beds. Special hospitals for tuberculosis were built by the insurance funds in Europe. In Latin America after 1939, many general hospitals were built by social security agencies specifically for insured persons.

Also in the late nineteenth century, the great technical developments in medicine led to much wider appreciation of the hospital as a place of choice for treatment of serious illness, regardless of a person's economic level. With asepsis, improvements in surgery, anesthesia, the rise of professional nursing, and other advances, hospitals became centers of medical science. Medical schools became increasingly affiliated with large hospitals or were even founded by hospitals.

Recognition of the infectiousness of tuberculosis and the possibilities of cure through prolonged bed rest gave rise to the sanitarium. To be economical, a tuberculosis sanitarium usually had to be quite large. Hence, the most practical type of sponsorship came from larger units of government—the province or the central national authority. The same applied in the nineteenth century to asylums for the insane, who had previously been confined in prisons with criminals.

Since the fifteenth century, European governments had had national hospitals for military men and sometimes police. Merchant mariners were also provided with special hospitals at the main ports of England, and the same was done in the United States after 1798. Later in the nineteenth century, some governments that built railroads set up hospitals for railroad workers. In the twentieth century, especially in the less developed countries, other government employees were provided with separate hospitals.

In the late nineteenth and early twentieth centuries, private industry also built hospitals for workers at isolated enterprises such as mining and lumbering locations. In the less developed countries of Latin America, Asia, and Africa, small private hospitals were established at sugar plantations, tea, and rubber estates, and other agricultural enterprises. After 1885, industrial injury compensation laws encouraged such construction, since these laws obligated employers to meet the medical costs of work injuries.

In the colonies of Asia and Africa, local government was weak or nonexistent, so that the hospitals were controlled by central government, first in the colonial capitals, then in other cities. When these European colonies became emancipated, the strong central control of public hospitals was usually maintained. Religious missions from Europe and the United States also established some rural hospitals; later these were often integrated into national hospital systems.

Finally, in the twentieth century, some hospitals have been established as purely commercial enterprises. Usually with the combined support of private physicians and wealthy families, these proprietary facilities have been built to serve wealthy or upper-middle-class families. Typically, these units are small but well provided with nursing personnel and modern equipment.

With these multiple origins, one can understand why today in most countries one sees hospitals under various forms of sponsorship or ownership. This has a major bearing on their mode of operation—their staffing, functions, and participation in planned regional health care systems.

Hospital Sponsorships

The mixture of hospital sponsorships in a country naturally depends on the relative impact of several historical streams we have just reviewed, as well as on the country's political structure. In the United States, with its strong free enterprise character, the general hospitals (which account for 95 percent of hospital admissions each year) are predominantly privately sponsored—whether church supported, voluntary nonprofit, or proprietary. Only about one-third of the general hospital beds are in governmental facilities, usually local units of government. However, in the United States, as is true of most countries, mental hospital beds are under government control. There are also substantial numbers of facilities of all types for special population groups (e.g., military veterans, soldiers, or American Indians) controlled by the federal government.

In a welfare state such as Sweden, the sponsorship picture is quite different. About 95 percent of all the beds, both general and mental, are in governmental hospitals. It is local units of government, equivalent to American counties, that own and operate them. Their boards of directors are appointed by locally elected officials. In France, where the welfare state ideology is somewhat less highly developed, about two-thirds of the general hospital beds and 70 percent of the total beds are governmentally owned; the balance are operated privately for profit. (It will be recalled that, after the French Revolution, the church-owned nonprofit hospitals were taken over by government.)

In 1948 Great Britain, although not a socialist country in the usual political sense, put almost all its hospitals under the control of the central Ministry of Health. The management of hospitals, however, has been until recently delegated to Regional Hospital Boards (fifteen in England and Wales). With the 1974 reorganization of the British National Health Service, responsibility has been even more decentralized to some ninety Area Health Authorities. The ultimate controls, however, are still vested in the central government. Almost every hospital, nevertheless, maintains a small fraction—usually less than 5 percent—of beds for purely private patients who pay supplemental fees to the hospital as well as the full charges of the physician. A good deal of controversy has been occurring recently about the social equity of this arrangement.

Turning to a transitional country, for example, Peru, we see a mixture of hospital sponsorships that reflect its national history. Since the Catholic church was a powerful force historically, the local boards of the *beneficencia* societies control 42 percent of the general hospital beds. (This is in spite of a substantial subsidy by government and their obligation to abide by certain governmental standards.) About 14 percent of the general beds are under the control of private industry or proprietary owners. The balance of 44 percent of the beds are government controlled, divided between the Ministry of Health and the social security institutes, there being two separate central authorities.

A transitional developing country in Asia such as Iran has a somewhat similar mixture of sponsorships. Considering total beds, 56 percent are sponsored by the central government, 32 percent by charitable nonprofit bodies, and 12 percent by proprietary owners. Considering general hospitals alone, however, it is 46 percent that are government controlled. In other words, for day-to-day medical care, the general hospitals mainly have been sponsored, as in Peru, by religious, charitable, or other nongovernmental bodies.

The more extremely underdeveloped countries of Africa display more predominantly governmental sponsorship of hospitals. In Togo, a former French colony, for example, the total supply of beds is very low, at about 1.5 per 1,000 population; practically all these beds, however, are under the control of the central government. In Uganda, a former British colony, the bed ratio is about the same, and of these beds nearly 70 percent are controlled by government. Nearly all the remainder are under nonprofit agencies, mainly religious missions. Indonesia, with fewer than 0.70 beds per 1,000 population, has 78 percent of them under government control; the balance are voluntary nonprofit.

Hospital sponsorship in the fully socialist countries, as one would expect, is 100 percent governmental. The degree of control by central government, as distinguished from local authorities, however, is much greater in countries such as the Soviet Union, Hungary, or Cuba than in the People's Republic of China or Yugoslavia.

We have not dwelled on the available supply of hospital beds in all these types of countries, but on the whole this varies with a country's per capita wealth and its political philosophy. The interplay of these two determinants is complex, and it is further complicated by the purposes for which hospital beds are used and the intensity of patient care. Thus, the wealthy United States, according to data reported by the World Health Organization, has a total of 7.5 beds per 1,000 population (as of 1971), of which about 4.0 are in general hospitals. Norway, a less affluent country, but supported by a strong welfare state ideology, has 13.1 total beds per 1,000 population. Czechoslovakia, much less affluent than the United States or Norway but with a fully socialist policy, has 10.1 beds per 1,000 population. Nevertheless, because of a shorter average length of stay, the United States has a higher rate of hospital admissions (158 per 1,000 population per year) than Norway (139 per 1,000). Czechoslovakia's admission rate is slightly higher than both at 164 per 1,000 population per year.

Brazil, a transitional country, has 3.8 total hospital beds per 1,000 population. Guatemala has 2.2 per 1,000. Severely underdeveloped countries, of course, have even fewer—0.33 beds per 1,000 in Ethiopia or 1.24 per 1,000 in Kenya.

For planning purposes, the optimal supply of hospital beds needed by each country has been a subject of study and debate everywhere. If there is an assured payment system, it seems that almost any additional hospital beds provided will tend to be used, up to a ceiling not yet determined. The ideal bed-population ratio obviously depends on the prevalence of disease or injury and the characteristics of the whole health care system. In many affluent countries, rising medical care costs have led in recent years to a judgment that the bed supply is excessive. In the poorer countries, the bed supply is still clearly less than the needs, even though improved transportation and education are usually required to enable the people to make better use of the beds available.

Types of Hospitals

By far the greatest proportion of admissions in any country are to general hospitals, which provide care for ordinary surgical or medical conditions, and usually for maternity cases as well. In many countries, however, there are separate institutions for maternity care, communicable diseases, and children. The economically more developed countries have tended to move away from these latter types and have used general hospitals for nearly all short-term or acute conditions.

Long-term disorders, on the other hand, are usually served in special hospitals in all types of country. This is especially true of mental disorders. Yet, as more has been learned about psychiatry, it has been feasible to admit even patients with psychiatric diagnoses to general hospitals for short-term treatment—usually less than thirty days. Mental hospitals in nearly all countries are poorly financed and typically provide a very low standard of care, even in the most affluent economies.

There is obviously an interplay among various types of hospitals with respect to the diagnoses of patients treated. If the general hospitals in a country, for example, customarily serve patients with acute infectious diseases, there will tend not to be separate hospitals for such cases. Similarly, if funds are readily available to construct hospitals for maternity care and for sick children, then the provision for such cases in general hospitals will be reduced.

To clarify these interrelations and also other influences on the types of hospitals in a country, we may look at the percentage distributions in Table 1. For the United States, as well as all the other countries except Brazil, well over half of all hospital beds are in general facilities. Mental institutions have almost half as many beds in the United States as the general hospitals. All the other types have only tiny percentages of bed resources, but the explanations differ. Tuberculosis beds were formerly a substantial share of the total, but over the past twenty years the incidence of this disease has been greatly reduced. Special hospitals for maternity and child cases are scarce because such patients are

TABLE 1   Types of Hospital: Percentage Distribution of Beds, by Type of Hospital in Five Countries, 1971

Type	Country				
	United States	Belgium	Nigeria	Brazil	Poland
General	62.1	57.0	83.2	39.7	59.1
Mental	32.1	33.0	4.3	23.6	15.9
Tuberculosis	1.1	3.0	0.8	6.9	10.1
Infectious disease	–	–	2.1	1.2	2.0
Leprosy	0.03	–	3.4	7.2	–
Maternity and children	0.4	–	3.9	16.6	3.9
Chronic and aged	2.2	7.0	–	0.8	8.8
Other special	2.0	–	2.4	4.7	0.3
Total	100.0	100.0	100.0	100.0	100.0
(number)	1,555,560	80,392	35,716	354,373	251,593
Beds per 1000 population	7.5	8.3	0.63	3.8	7.7

Source: Derived from *World Health Statistics Annual: Health Personnel and Hospital Establishments*, World Health Organization, Geneva, 1975.

conventionally served in general hospitals. Leprosy cases occupy only a minuscule fraction of the beds. The proportion of only 2.2 percent of beds for the chronically ill and aged must be explained differently. In the United States a very large complement of private nursing homes has developed for these patients; in fact, there are more beds in such intermediate or extended care facilities than in all the general hospitals. But nursing homes—and these may provide varying intensities of technical service—are not licensed as hospitals; hence, they are not included in these statistics. Furthermore, many general hospitals have a sizable proportion of their beds occupied by the chronically ill or even maintain special wards for such patients.

In Belgium, which is considered among the welfare state type of countries, the distribution of general and mental beds is roughly parallel to that in the United States. The proportion of beds for the chronically ill and aged, however, is three times higher. This can hardly be explained by the slightly higher proportion of aged persons in that country; it is owing rather to the fact that the private nursing home industry in Belgium is much smaller. The higher proportion of tuberculosis beds in Belgium similarly does not reflect a higher prevalence of that disease but rather a tendency to maintain fewer beds in general hospitals for TB patients.

In the underdeveloped countries, for example, Nigeria, the mix of beds is strikingly different. The proportion of beds for mental patients is far lower than in any of the other four countries. This is not because mental patients are placed in general hospitals (except on rare occasions) but because, owing to the over-all weakness of hospital resources in this impoverished nation there is little identification of mental disorder as such. Persons with mental disturbances simply stay with their families and communities without being classified as sick. Similarly, the tiny fraction of beds for tuberculosis is deceptive; this disease is of high prevalence in Nigeria. Most cases, however, are simply not identified; those that are diagnosed are treated either at home or sometimes in general hospitals. The relatively large portion of beds devoted to leprosy (3.4 percent), on the other hand, reflects not only the high prevalence of this disease but the social attitude that such patients must be isolated.

In Brazil, to illustrate the transitional countries, the proportion of beds in general hospitals seems remarkably small. This is owing mainly, however, to the existence of many special hospitals for maternity care and sick children—16.6 percent of the total. If this percentage is added to that for the general hospital beds, it comes to 56.3 percent or nearly the same proportion as in Belgium, which lacks any special maternity and child care facilities. In Brazil it has been relatively easy to raise funds for the hospital care of mothers and children because of social attitudes. The relatively high proportions of beds devoted to both tuberculosis and leprosy reflect a high prevalence of both of these chronic infectious diseases in Brazil, as well as policy decisions to isolate these cases.

In socialist Poland, the relatively low proportion of beds for mental patients, compared with the other industrialized countries, may be due to various reasons. Socialist ideologists might claim that it means a lower occurrence of mental disorders in such a society; on the other hand, it may simply mean that such patients are less frequently recognized as being ill, or it may mean that they are kept at home. The exceptionally high proportion of beds for tuberculosis (10.1 percent) means not so much a high prevalence of this disease (the mortality rate is not much higher than that in the United States or Belgium) but rather a policy decision to hospitalize all such cases. Also, the high proportion of beds for the aged and chronically ill reflects a policy of putting such patients in special hospitals as distinguished from general hospitals or intermediate nursing homes.

There are many more special features to hospital facilities than summarized here. The size of hospitals is an important characteristic that influences their functions. The distribution of hospital sizes differs greatly among countries, more large-capacity facilities being established in the more urbanized countries. The time of a building's construction is also relevant. European hospitals, for obvious historical reasons, tend to be older than those in the United States or in the more recently developing countries. In older hospitals, different structural styles were followed, with more separate pavilions than in the consolidated new facilities. Among chronic disease hospitals there may be special facilities for rheumatic disorders built adjacent to mineral springs or spas. There may also be specially designed institutions for the blind or deaf. Mental hospitals vary from colonies of many small cottages to huge prison-like fortresses; in Israel there is, indeed, an ancient fort serving as a mental hospital. In a word, hospitals are highly sensitive to the time and place that they are built, the resources available, political settings, social attitudes, and the functions they are to serve.

Hospital Functions and Trends

Everywhere hospitals provide bed care for the seriously sick, but increasingly in most countries they have been carrying out a wider range of functions. More attention is being given everywhere to outpatient services—the diagnosis and treatment of the ambulatory patient. Larger hospitals, especially in the more economically advanced and in the socialist countries, are devoting increasing attention to research and the education of health personnel. This is quite aside from the broadening range of diagnostic and treatment services for inpatients that are in step with the advances of medical science.

In free enterprise countries (and some welfare states, such as Japan or Belgium) where there is great local autonomy of hospitals, innovative ideas may be readily developed, but there is great unevenness in applying them. The concept of organized home care that originated in the United States for the care of certain chronically ill patients demonstrates this. Although it has been effectively applied in certain large city institutions, most American hospitals have no such programs. On the other hand, in Great Britain, with its National Health Service, there is greater uniformity of application of any policy that is promoted. For example, the outpatient department of almost every British hospital is well developed; by contrast, the great majority of American hospitals have only an emergency room and no organized outpatient clinics at all.

In some countries, the broad concept of the hospital serving as the center for all health services in an area has special significance. This is the philosophy of the Soviet Union's hospitals, where the hospital director is theoretically responsible for all health activities in the surrounding area, including the ambulatory and preventive services. Thus, nearby health centers are regarded as administrative satellites of the hospital. The same concept was applied in the original formulation of the National Health Service in Chile. In many underdeveloped and transitional countries, this policy is implemented in varying degrees.

As centers for education, large hospitals have played an important part in the training of doctors for centuries. More recently they have become increasingly involved in postgraduate education, offering regular conferences and meetings on problems of clinical medicine. Their role in training other health personnel has also been expanding. Nursing education started in hospitals about a century ago, and the training of other types of allied health worker has grown steadily. In North America since World War II, nursing education has been gradually being transfered to community colleges, with only the field practice aspects conducted in affiliated hospitals. In Europe and the other continents, however, the general hospitals are still the principal locale for nursing education, as well as for the training of laboratory technicians, physiotherapists, and other types of personnel. Cuba has a policy of regarding every hospital as a training center for various types of middle-level health worker, such as nursing assistants.

Until quite recently, the general trend has been for more and more of the total health services to be rendered within hospital walls. Childbirth, for a major example, was an event that properly took place at home fifty years ago in almost all countries. Today, in all industrialized countries, over 90 percent of deliveries are done in hospitals (even when done by midwives, associated traditionally with childbirths in the home). In the poorer, developing countries, the effort is also being made to increase steadily the proportion of babies delivered in hospitals. Such arrangements have led to a great reduction in maternal and perinatal mortality, especially when home conditions are unsanitary. The same increased tendency to use the hospital is seen everywhere for cases of pneumonia, heart failure, strokes, or other nonsurgical diagnoses that were attended in previous decades at home.

Elaborate diagnostic workups of complex cases are done in hospitals, largely because of the difficulty of carrying out numerous procedures on an ambulatory basis. The range of possible therapies that can be done only in hospitals has steadily widened—open-heart surgery, kidney dialyses, organ transplants, rehabilitation of severely disabled patients, or short-term treatment of acute mental disorders. The relative intensity of service to virtually all types of case—the numbers of tests as well as therapeutic procedures—has continually increased. As a result, an enlarging share, as much as 40 to 60 percent of the total, of the money spent for health service in most countries has been allocated to hospital care.

This great proportion of total funds going to hospitals is often at the expense of adequate expenditures for ambulatory and preventive services. Elaborate therapy for a single patient in the hospital may require money that, if applied to community preventive services, could save scores of lives. Although such imbalances may be seen in all countries, they are especially regrettable in the poorest underdeveloped countries where the total funds for health service are so inadequate and the potentials for disease prevention so great. Yet the dramatic aspects and advanced scientific technology of hospital service are often regarded as more politically attractive than simple preventive services, especially in rural villages.

The complexity of hospital service varies with the wealth of countries, and even between regions within a nation. In the United States and Canada, the staffing and equipment of hospitals tends to be more elaborate than in most European countries, both Western and Eastern. European hospitals are, in turn, much more highly developed than the average hospital in Latin America or India, which are, in turn, more complex than the average hospital in Africa. This can be quantified in the ratio of hospital personnel per patient. In an American hospital of 200-bed capacity, there would be about 500 personnel or 2.5 per bed; in a European hospital of this size about 1.5 to 2.0 per bed; in a Latin American hospital about 1;0; and in an African hospital about 0.5 per bed. With such gradations in staffing, the rapidity of management of cases is roughly proportional. Thus, the average duration of stay in hospitals is usually longer as staffing becomes weaker. A gall bladder surgery case in New York, for example, would average about eight days of hospitalization (varying with the patient's age and other factors), in Amsterdam about twelve days, in Bogotá about fifteen days, and in Nairobi about twenty days. Other factors, such as the patient's home environment, also influence length of stay in hospitals, and even in the same country the average stay tends to be longer in rural areas than in cities. In any event, a shorter average stay per case means that a given hospital can admit more patients per year than the same size hospital with longer average stays.

In many countries, the enlarging share of the health care dollar being absorbed by hospitals is generating reactions. More attention is being devoted to health centers where proper treatment and preventive services can be given to ambulatory patients. In the United States, where the cost of a day of hospital care has come to exceed $100, "surgicenters" for performance of relatively minor surgical procedures on outpatients are being developed to avoid these high expenditures. In the larger cities of many countries, organized home care programs are being conducted by some hospitals to reduce the hospital stays of chronically ill patients.

Preventive services have, on the whole, been only weakly developed as a hospital function. There are general hospitals operated in Japan by agricultural cooperatives (118 of them) that are rather unusual in offering programs of health education and screening tests for incipient chronic disease in rural populations. Many hospitals in the Soviet Union and other socialist countries also provide health education to patients and to visitors. The most frequent preventive activity of hospitals on a world-wide basis is conducting maternal and child health clinics in their outpatient departments. In general, however, hospitals look to public health agencies to offer preventive service, while they concentrate their efforts on treatment of severely sick or injured patients.

Hospital Administration and Financing

The pattern of internal administration of a hospital depends to a large extent on its sponsorship or ownership. If it is sponsored by a religious body or a nonsectarian voluntary association, the top authority is typically vested in a board of directors. On this board are typically persons who have made large donations to the cost of building the hospital or their descendants and other persons of social prominence in the area. Board members or trustees usually select their own successors. These self-perpetuating bodies establish the top policy of the hospital, usually within certain constraints of law or regulation. They appoint the personnel to administer and work in the hospital and may establish rules about the type of patients to be admitted.

The concept of hospital boards as governing bodies has been so widely established that many government-sponsored hospitals also have them. The members of such boards, however, are typically appointed by an elected body, such as a County Council in Sweden. Requirements for board membership may be defined by law, as in France, where, for example, an intermediate hospital board must contain nine members—the town mayor as chairman, two appointees of the municipal council, one appointee of the general council of the *département,* two representatives of the social security program (which finances a major share of hospital operation), one representative of the hospital doctors, one representative of doctors in the local community, and a citizen interested in hospital affairs.

In Great Britain with its National Health Service, there have been until recently Regional Hospital Boards that were responsible for all the hospitals in a region of two or three million people. The board was chosen by the national Minister of Health, and it, in turn, appointed a Hospital Management Committee to administer each hospital. In transitional countries with predominantly governmental hospitals, such as Chile or Malaysia, there are no hospital boards at all. Each government facility simply has a director in charge, and he reports to a zone or provincial health officer. This sort of hierarchy of administative controls is found also in the mainly public hospitals of the underdeveloped countries of Africa. It is the pattern also in most socialist countries.

When this pyramidal pattern of hospital authority prevails, there are sometimes local advisory bodies composed of residents of the area. In Malaysia these are called Boards of Visitors. In the Soviet Union, the local Communist Party organization exercises a certain supervision over the hospitals. In the People's Republic of China, each hospital—like each factory or school—is headed by a Revolutionary Committee representing the various personnel on the hospital staff.

The day-to-day management of most hospitals in the United States is usually delegated by the board of directors to a hospital administrator. The administrator, with various assistant administrators, is responsible for all the departments—nursing service, business affairs, food and laundry, diagnostic laboratories, the pharmacy, housekeeping, and so on. The medical staff in different clinical divisions (surgery, medicine, obstetrics, etc.) are theoretically also responsible to the board of directors through the administrator, although in most American voluntary hospitals, the doctors, being mainly engaged as independent private practitioners rather than as hospital employees, relate directly to the board.

In the majority of countries, however, the principal executive in most hospitals is a physician, serving as medical director. He is typically assisted by a business manager or a financial officer and also by a nursing director. The doctors on the hospital staff, being mainly on salaries, are under the authority of the medical director, although professional tradition grants them great independence in the clinical management of patients. This concept of medical leadership at the top is found in most of the welfare state countries, in the transitional and underdeveloped countries, and in most of the socialist countries within the government-sponsored hospitals that predominate in nearly all these settings. There are some hospitals, however, in most nonsocialist countries with open medical staffs, where outside doctors can take their private patients. In these, the American pattern is more often found, that is, a nonmedical administrator responsible for everything except clinical decisions on patient care.

This American scheme of hospital administration has been described as having two lines of authority—one managerial and the other medical. Since the jurisdictions of these two sectors are often difficult to define, there are frequent controversies. There is a very high turnover of hospital administrators in the United States, usually because of disputes with the private medical staff or because of becoming caught in crossfire between the doctors and the board of directors. In British hospitals, a modus vivendi has frequently been found by establishing a trio of top management—doctor, manager, and head nurse (or matron). Each has his or her own domain of responsibility, and they work closely together. However, in most countries, as noted, a physician exercises top authority because he commands most respect in the hospital. Moreover, trained hospital administrators who are not doctors are quite rare outside of North America. In the underdeveloped and transitional countries, furthermore, the supply of doctors is so low that the medical director may also give clinical service in the hospital, especially if it is a small facility in a rural region.

Regarding the physical layout of hospitals, the degree of privacy accorded to patients tends to depend on national wealth. In the free enterprise and welfare state countries, private or semiprivate rooms with only two or three patients are the general rule. In the other three types of countries, larger wards with about ten to thirty patients are most common. Still, these predominant patterns are by no means universal in each type of country. In wealthy America, there are still numerous public hospitals for the poor with thirty-bed wards, especially if these institutions are quite old. On the other hand, in Latin America and in Iran, there are newly built hospitals under the sponsorship of social security agencies, in which the largest ward contains only three or four beds. The welfare states of Western Europe and the socialist countries of Eastern Europe have attached such importance to hospital care that facilities constructed in recent years usually emphasize very personalized attention, with rooms containing no more than two or three beds.

The older hospitals in Europe and elsewhere tend to have very decentralized or fragmented architectural design. Typically spread out and lacking elevators, they have separate buildings or pavilions for different types of patient—surgical or medical, men, women or children, and so on. It is common for small separate laboratories and pharmacies to be attached to each section. With modern architecture and the consolidation of room space in one structure served by elevators, it has been feasible to design facilities with centralized support services for laboratory tests, drugs, medical records, and so on. More recently built hospitals are also characterized by larger outpatient quarters, since hospital functions have become so extended in the field of ambulatory care.

In almost all countries, the financial support of hospital services has become more collectivized than that of other components of health care. Even in the free enterprise setting of the United States, the major share of hospital costs is now met by insurance, either voluntary or social (governmental). Another large portion of hospital costs for the indigent or special groups like veterans is covered by public revenues. Only a small fraction of American hospital financing today, approximately 10 percent, comes from purely private payments.

In the welfare state systems, the social insurance programs pay nearly all the costs of hospital care except in certain countries. Sweden is one such exception where, owing to long historical precedent, the county governments bear the bulk of hospital costs. Only about 10 percent is contributed by social insurance, although it pays nearly all out-of-hospital medical costs. Also, in the British National Health Service, hospital costs are borne predominantly by general revenues. Canada illustrates a pattern in which about half of hospital financing is derived from federal general revenues and the other half from various sorts of provincial taxes. Some provinces raise the money through social insurance mechanisms, others through provincial general revenues, and others through special sales taxes. In Germany, France, Denmark, Belgium, Italy, and Japan, social insurance bears the main burden of hospital costs.

In the transitional countries, with their public hospitals for the poor and special social security hospitals for the steadily employed minority of the population, costs are borne by general revenues and social insurance, respectively. The charitable or religiously sponsored hospitals also get most of their operating funds from general revenues, with a fraction coming from philanthropy, rent from lands bequested, or interest from investment of previous donations. In the underdeveloped countries, central revenues bear nearly all the costs of public hospitals, which contain the great majority of beds. In both these types of developing country, there are small private hospitals for the well-to-do that are financed by fees from patients.

Finally, in the socialist countries, hospitals are financed simply by general governmental revenues. The detailed fiscal mechanism in these hospitals, as well as in many government hospitals of the other types of country, is much simpler than that prevailing for most hospitals in the United States or some welfare states such as France or Belgium. Periodic global payments cover the full cost of operating each hospital, based on its total budget. Sometimes called prospective reimbursement, this method contrasts sharply with the payment to hospitals on the basis of charges for each patient day of care or even for each specific in-patient service, such as the laboratory tests, medications, and the like. The latter method gives the hospital incentives to maximize patient days or units of service and, therefore, readily escalates over-all costs. The former method gives incentives to economy and to prudent use of all services. On the other hand, government must exercise surveillance to be sure that standards are met and that patients are not underserviced.

Regionalization of Health Facilities

As medical science has advanced, hospitals everywhere have been faced with the problem of how much technology they should attempt to encompass in their service. Can one expect every hospital to offer the full range of technical ser-

vices? Economies could obviously be achieved if expensive diagnostic and treatment procedures for conditions occurring infrequently in a population could be
concentrated in large centralized facilities of a geographic region, whereas simpler
resources for handling common conditions could be made available in every hospital. Then, if a rare, complex disorder occurs in a person living in an isolated
rural area, he could be transported to the central facility; for common and simpler conditions, he could be treated in a local hospital nearby.

The planning of networks of hospitals along such lines has been defined as
regionalization. The concept has been appreciated in almost every country, but
its implementation has not been easy everywhere. Both the initial construction
of facilities and their subsequent functioning are involved. Even if buildings are
rationally planned according to regionalized principles, decisions on the care of
individual patients may not always be made correspondingly. Moreover, functional regionalization also means a flow of information from the center peripherally, to continually upgrade the knowledge of more isolated health personnel.
This requires effort and expenditures. It presumes some sort of organization of
all the resources in the geographic region.

In free enterprise United States, the regionalization concept has been only
weakly applied, since the vast majority of hospitals are independent and autonomous. In 1947 a federal program for subsidizing needed hospital construction
required that all building projects fit into a regionalized master plan drawn up in
each state. Such projects, however, affected only about one-quarter of the hospitals. Moreover, since private medical practice prevails and the medical staff
organization in most hospitals is relatively loose and informal, little was done
to implement a two-way flow of patients and medical information among the
hospitals in a region. In 1966 new legislation on regional medical programs to
treat patients with heart disease, cancer, and stroke (the leading causes of death)
fostered educational programs reaching out from medical schools to peripheral
hospitals but did nothing on systematic referral of patients. Certain subsystems
in America, such as that of the federal Veterans Administration hospitals, apply
regionalized concepts for their special population of patients.

In the European welfare state countries, regionalization is generally more
fully applied, insofar as all new hospital construction (not solely that which is
subsidized by national grants) must be approved by the national government.
In France, with its centralized hospital legislation, the equipping, staffing, and
operation of facilities (with graded responsibilities in networks around medical
schools) have been systematically done. In Norway, although both construction
and operational responsibilities are vested in the counties, the payments for care
by the social insurance system exercise fiscal controls over the staffing of each
hospital. Great Britain, with its Regional Health Authorities (formerly Regional
Hospital Boards), has a firm administrative basis for regionalization, since important decisions on the affairs of all hospitals in a region of two or three million

people are made by a single body. Duplications or gaps in services can thus be avoided.

In the transitional countries of Latin America and the Middle East, regionalization principles are well applied within the subsystems of social security agencies or ministries of health or even of the charitable hospital societies. However, there may be a serious lack of coordination across these subsystems. Only in Chile has the Ministry of Health been successful in establishing zone or regional authorities under which all facilities in the jurisdication are coordinated according to a regional plan. A movement toward achievement of such coordinated plans under central government control, however, is seen in almost all these countries.

The underdeveloped countries of Africa and parts of Asia demonstrate well the regionalization idea in its theory. With severe poverty of resources, however, there are many gaps in the networks of facilities required. The central hospitals in the capital cities nearly always have been built; these are often affiliated with medical schools and they meet the personal needs of families in the small middle class or the power elite. In the secondary towns serving rural regions there tend to be serious hospital deficiencies.

In the socialist countries, regionalization of hospitals has been most fully achieved. With substantially centralized planning, the role and resources of each institution are explicitly defined. Ambulance services for transporting patients have been well developed, even though personally owned automobiles are in very short supply (as a result of deliberate planning policies). With all doctors and other medical personnel on government salaries, there are no monetary incentives to give a service in a hospital not properly staffed and equipped for it. The personal pride of a surgeon in a small rural facility may lead him to operate on a patient who should be transferred to a central facility, but this sort of deviation is rare. It would not long withstand surveillance from higher levels.

In spite of these differences among countries, the world-wide movement is clearly toward principles of hospital regionalization. In the interests of both quality and economy and to equalize access to needed services for all persons, wherever they may live, regionalization is the obvious answer. Its implementation requires centralized planning, rather than the proud sovereignty of individual hospitals. The smooth relationship among the parts of an organization, which is the hallmark of good internal hospital administration, should be paralleled in geographic regions by a systematic two-way flow of patients and technical consultation to meet optimally the health needs of large populations.

Ideally, regionalization involves more than the care of hospital patients; it involves ambulatory services as well. Administratively branched from the hospital at each echelon should be properly staffed ambulatory facilities for both treatment and preventive service. Their mode of existence and development in different types of country will be considered in the next section.

Health Centers and Other Facilities

Strictly speaking, the office of every private health practitioner (physician, dentist, optometrist, and so on) is a small health facility. When several auxiliary personnel work with the health practitioner, the establishment requires more organization and management. A private group medical practice, with several physicians and others working together, requires still more planning, organization, supervision, records, and so on.

Corresponding facilities for teams of health personnel serving the ambulatory person have been established by governments or other social bodies throughout the world under the term *health center*. This term, and the concept of a structure with several rooms for defined purposes, was applied originally to buildings devoted essentially to preventive services in the early twentieth century. Much earlier, separate dispensaries, as they were called, had been set up in cities for ambulatory treatment of the poor outside of hospitals. However, these were typically very humble places—perhaps a room or two in the basement of a public building or space in a converted private house.

The concept of the health center as an establishment combining primary medical care by general practitioners and organized preventive services was first formulated in England in 1920. The Consultative Council on Medical and Allied Services, under the chairmanship of Lord Dawson of Penn, recommended in the Dawson Report that a network of such units should be set up throughout the country as an improved method of providing integrated primary ambulatory services. For secondary care by specialists, either outpatient or inpatient, the person would be referred to a hospital.

The opposition of the private medical profession killed this idea in England, as it did similar ideas in the United States in the 1920s. A politically acceptable formulation at that time, however, was to provide health centers devoted to various types of preventively oriented services—infant health stations, venereal disease or tuberculosis clinics, immunizations, the offices of sanitarians and public health nurses, adult classes on nutrition or hygiene, and so on. In 1926 a model health center with such preventive purposes was built in Ceylon as part of the British Colonial Medical Service. Several such units were established also in large cities of the United States to house the preventive programs of various voluntary health agencies as well as the offices of local health departments.

Health centers on the Dawson Report model that combined primary treatment and prevention were actually first launched in the Soviet Union soon after the Russian Revolution of 1917. With no obstruction from private entrepreneurial interests, networks of health centers were built as the logical first echelon of health service, leading to polyclinics with specialists, to intermediate hospitals, and then to large medical centers. In the 1940s, this idea came to be widely emulated throughout the developing continents.

Today in the United States, most facilities defined as health centers are still structures to house departments of public health or district units of such departments in the larger cities. Health centers providing integrated primary care are typically limited to selected population groups. Largely as a response to the urban riots of the 1960s, neighborhood health centers were built in the heart of poverty districts under various types of governmental auspices. Such centers numbered about 200 by 1975. Also after World War II, labor health centers were constructed by several unions or labor-management trust funds to provide prepaid diagnostic, treatment, and preventive services to union members and their families. Private group practice clinics, often in impressive structures, have multiplied to the point that they now involve about 20 percent of American doctors in clinical work, but the majority of doctors are still in individual private practice.

In Great Britain, the early plans for the National Health Service in 1946 contemplated a large network of health centers in which general practitioners remaining in private practice would rent space alongside public health nurses, social workers, and other personnel employed by local government. For twenty years, the concept was implemented only in a few places. Then in the late 1960s, the interest of British general practitioners to work in such settings increased, perhaps owing to the fact that private group clinics of general practitioners had been rapidly growing. Starting in the new towns, where there were no established doctors, local government authorities built small health centers in which general practitioners found it convenient to rent quarters. The proximity of community nurses, social workers, and sometimes laboratory technicians facilitated their clinical work. By 1975, there were 300 to 400 of such health centers in England and Scotland, and the numbers were continuing to expand.

Other welfare state countries of Western Europe are developing health centers on a more limited basis. In France, groups of private doctors, both general practitioners and specialists, have established clinics where preventive services are emphasized but treatment is also given. Fees are charged to patients, who are reimbursed by the social security program, but unlike the custom in most private practice, the fees are always under the ceiling of the official fee schedule. Similar ambulatory facilities under the term of *polyclinics* have been established in Belgium by the local mutual societies. In Japan, where the private medical profession is especially powerful, a network of government health centers is still limited to the provision of preventive services.

In the less developed countries of both the transitional and the underdeveloped types, health centers are widely available. They are the principal channel for provision of scientific primary health care, especially in the rural regions. In the social security programs of the transitional countries, health centers or polyclinics, rather than private medical offices, are the conventional settings for providing general as well as specialty medical care. In the underdeveloped countries, health centers are staffed mainly by allied health personnel, whereas the relatively few government doctors are stationed mainly in hospitals. It is customary in Africa for female assistant nurses to give the preventive services in health centers, whereas male medical assistants and dispensers give the curative services.

It is in the socialist countries that health centers are the most highly developed mode for the provision of ambulatory care to the total population. Since private medical and dental practice has almost died out, nearly all ambulatory services are provided in health centers, polyclinics, or in the outpatient departments of hospitals. In all these facilities, there are physicians along with allied personnel. For very small health stations in thinly settled rural areas of the Soviet Union, the staffing may consist only of *feldshers* or *feldsher*-midwives. In rural China also, at the level of the production brigade (500 to 3,000 people), a small clinic room provides space for one or more "barefoot doctors." At the higher level of the Chinese commune (20,000 to 60,000 people), however, there are health centers staffed by fully trained doctors.

In all five types of country, the administrative structure of health centers is nearly always quite simple, with a physician in charge or, in his absence, usually the senior medical auxiliary. Perhaps the major exception is in the neighborhood health center that emerged in the United States in the 1960s, where racial strife led to a major movement for consumer control. One expression of this trend has been the election of citizen boards of directors for many of these units and the designation of nonmedical administrators as the chief executives. In the rural areas of all types of country, it is common for health centers to contain small pharmacies from which drugs are dispensed to patients on the spot. Laboratory equipment for a few simple tests is also usually available.

Besides hospitals and health centers, there are several other types of facility for special components of health care in all countries. Best known is the independent pharmacy where drugs as well as related medical supplies are sold. Most hospitals have their own pharmacy units, as do many health centers, but in the larger cities of all five types of country there are separate pharmacies where drugs can be purchased by the ambulatory patient.

In the free enterprise countries, where control over private commerce has been very limited, pharmacies have been established widely as small business units. In the cities, there are usually so many that competition has been too great to permit them all to be economically viable from drug sales alone. As a result, the typical drug store has widened its offerings to include many other products—cosmetics, candy, soap, photographic supplies, tobacco products, clocks, and all sorts of sundries. Large corporations operate chains of multipurpose drug stores, with short-order food counters, stationery departments, children's toys, and many other items. In these settings, the pharmacist may spend only a small fraction of his time compounding or dispensing drugs.

In the welfare state countries, permits to establish pharmacies are often more restricted, and those set up are essentially devoted to the distribution of drugs, which not only protects the competitive position of licensed pharmacists, but also conserves their time more strictly for the object of their training. In Norway, for example, certain urban districts are deemed by the central government to be fully saturated with private pharmacies; a new pharmacy graduate may work in those districts only by purchasing an existing unit or being employed in it. A much more scientific and professional atmosphere characterizes these pharmacies than one finds in the United States.

Private pharmacies in the transitional countries are numerous in the main cities. As in the United States and Australia, they sell all sorts of commodities. In the small towns, they are often combined with general stores that sell food, liquor, and so on. In the underdeveloped countries, pharmacies are found only in the cities, although some drug compounds may be sold by grocery stores in small towns. In countries of Asia, such as the Philippines or Malaysia, many special shops are operated by Chinese herbalists, who freely prescribe for the patient when told his symptoms, as well as dispensing the remedy. In fact, dispensing is so closely associated with prescribing in the Orient that in Japan, although it is a highly developed country, the average private physician dispenses most of the drugs ordered for his patient. The same practice is found in Oriental city-states such as Singapore and Hong Kong.

In the socialist countries of Eastern Europe, all pharmacies are operated by the ministries of health. They are governmental facilities in the same sense as hospitals or health centers. Still, the patient must pay a share of the cost for most drugs (at low, controlled prices) except those for serious chronic disease, such as insulin for diabetes or digitalis for serious heart disease, and drugs for special categories of persons, such as pensioners or veterans. In Cuba, after the 1959 revolution, many superfluous city pharmacies were closed down, and new ones were set up in the small towns.

The laboratory is another type of facility that is usually an integral part of a hospital or health center but that in the free enterprise countries and some welfare states may operate as an independent establishment. Private pathologists or chemists may operate laboratories to perform tests for the private ambulatory patients of many doctors in an area.

Blood banks are typically units within larger hospitals in all types of country. In the less affluent countries, they are usually organized on a regional basis, with one facility serving several others around it and transporting needed blood by ambulance.

A complete inventory of health facilities must, finally, include clinics attached to other general establishments, such as factories, schools, or prisons. Such clinics are common in the industrialized (both free enterprise and welfare state) and also in the socialist countries; they are rare in the transitional and underdeveloped countries. In the main, the existence of these units and their adequacy relate to the establishment's size. In large establishments, they are often well developed. Small factories or schools cannot usually support separate health facilities and must use the resources of the general community.

Readings

Bell, John F., *The Family in the Hospital: Lessons from Developing Countries,* Washington, D.C.: U.S. Government Printing Office, 1970.

Berfenstam, R., "Cross-national Comparative Studies on Hospital Use," *World Hospitals, 9*:143-149 (October 1973).

Bravo, A. L. and A. P. Ruderman, *Costs and Utilization of Ministry and Social Security Medical Care Facilities in Latin America,* Washington, D.C.: Pan American Health Organization, 1966.

Bridgman, Robert F., *The Rural Hospital,* Geneva: World Health Organization, 1955.

———, *Hospital Utilization: An International Study,* Geneva: World Health Organization, 1976.

Brotherston, J. H. F., "The Use of the Hospital: Review of Research in the United Kingdom," *Medical Care, 1*:142-150, 225-231 (1963).

Byer, M. A. et al., "The Role of the Health Centre in an Integrated Health Programme in a Developing Country," *Medical Care, 4*:26-29 (January-March, 1966).

Dixon, C. W., "Regional Medical Planning in New Zealand," *New Zealand Medical Journal, 69*:371-374 (1969).

Dodu, Silas R. A., "The Hospital and the Pattern of Medical Practice in Ghana," *Ghana Medical Journal, 7*:96-99 (1968).

Engel, Arthur, *The Swedish Regionalized Hospital System,* Stockholm: National Board of Health, 1967;

Glaser, William A., *Social Settings and Medical Organization,* New York: Atherton, 1970.

Grant, John B., "Health Centers and Regionalization," *American Journal of Public Health, 43*:9-13 (January 1953).

Halevi, H. S., "Patterns of Hospitalization in England and Israel," *British Journal of Preventive and Social Medicine, 23*:196-202 (1969).

Hastings, J. E. F., *The Community Health Centre in Canada,* Ottawa: Information Canada, 1972.

Hogarth, James and T. E. Chester, "Health and Hospital Services in Denmark, Norway, and Sweden: A Comparative Analysis," *The Hospital, 56*:912-919 (November-December 1960).

International Hospital Federation, *The Changing Role of the Hospital in a Changing World,* London, 1963.

International Hospital Federation, *The Hospital Services of Europe,* London, 1966.

Leavell, Hugh R., "Regionalization of Health Services: An Examination of the

Regionalization Concept and W.H.O.'s Possible Role," Geneva: World Health Organization (processed), 1969.

Lembcke, Paul, "Hospital Efficiency—A Lesson from Sweden," *Hospitals, 33*: 34-48 (April 1959).

Llewelyn-Davies, R. and H. M. C. Macaulay, *Hospital Planning and Administration*, Geneva: World Health Organization, Monograph Series No. 54, 1966.

Reed, L. S. and W. Carr, "Utilization and Cost of General Hospital Care: Canada and the United States, 1948-1966," *Social Security Bulletin, 31*:12-20 (1968).

Roemer, Milton I., "The Impact of Hospitals on the Practice of Medicine in Europe and America," *Hospitals, 37*:61-64 (November 1963).

———, *Evaluation of Community Health Centeres*, Geneva: World Health Organization, Public Health Papers No. 48, 1972.

Roemer, Milton I. and Jay W. Friedman, "The World Scene in Doctor-Hospital Relations" in *Doctors in Hospitals: Medical Staff Organization and Hospital Performance*, Baltimore: Johns Hopkins Press, 1971.

Sigerist, Henry E., "An Outline of the Development of the Hospital," *Bulletin of the Institute of the History of Medicine, 4*:573-581 (July 1936).

Simpson, J., R. G. Thomas, H. N. Willard, and H. J. Bakst, *Custom and Practice in Medical Care, Comparative Study of Two Hospitals in Arbroath, Scotland, U.K., and Waterville, Maine, U.S.A.*, London: Oxford University Press, 1968.

Somers, H. M. and A. R. Somers, *Medicare and the Hospitals*, Washington, D.C.: Brookings Institution, 1967.

Spruyt, Dirk J., "Ethipoia's Health Center Program—Its Impact on Community Health," *Ethiopian Medical Journal, 5*:7-14 (January 1971).

World Health Organization, Expert Committee on Organization of Medical Care, *Role of Hospitals in Programmes of Community Health Protection*, Geneva: WHO Technical Report Series No. 122, 1957.

———, *Report of Expert Committee on Hospital Administration*, Geneva: WHO Technical Report Series No. 395, 1968.

6

DELIVERY OF MEDICAL CARE

Previous chapters have examined the methods of economic support for health
services and the types of resources, both manpower and physical facilities,
developed to provide such services around the world. In these discussions, we
inevitably said or implied how health personnel do their work. Here we will
look more closely at the various manners in which medical care is provided or
delivered in different national settings. This will involve, first, consideration
of primary (first contact) health care and the doctor-patient relationship. Second, we will look at the world-wide trend to specialization and the forms it
takes in different countries. Along with this the ways that doctors and others
work in hospitals are discussed. Third, the closely related methods of paying
the doctor and these methods' influence on performance must be considered.
Fourth, there are special problems of urban-rural distribution of health care in
all countries, and we will review how these have been tackled. Fifth, we will
consider delivery of certain types of health care that have often led to special
programs, such as mental health service, rehabilitation of the disabled, and dental
care. This chapter focuses on medical treatment, and the next one will examine
organized programs of prevention.

Primary Health Care

In every system of health services, there is some person to whom the patient,
whether sick or well, turns first for help. Strictly speaking, primary health care
includes both the initial response to the patient with a complaint—treatment or
referral—and preventive services given to the person who is presumably well.
Personal preventive services, however, will be considered later.

    An effective personal relationship between the patient and the doctor (or,
more broadly, the healer) has long been recognized as an important component

of good medical care. The patient entrusts himself to the doctor, and to do so, disclosing fully his intimate feelings and symptoms, he must have confidence in the doctor's integrity, ability, and concern. Ultimately, the relationship must be one-to-one, but as we will see, the over-all pattern of delivery of medical care in different settings may involve groups of doctors as well as third parties for financing. There are many social reasons for this, and one of the challenges in all patterns of delivery of health care is to maintain agreeable personal relationships, even though much social organization may be necessary to assure the patient financial access to the doctor and to maintain the quality of work of the doctor or other primary care provider.

It has sometimes been implied that the existence of any third party, such as a health insurance program or a government agency, constitutes interference in the patient-doctor relationship. Although it is possible that this is so, the predominant effect has been quite the opposite—namely, that collectivized methods of economic support generally facilitate access of the patient to the doctor, so that the two can achieve a relationship in the first place. On a world level, there is no doubt that poverty, with inability to pay qualified doctors or other healers, has been the major obstruction to the development of sound personal relationships in sickness care. More than money is obviously necessary, but we will see how sound and satisfactory patient-doctor relations can be attained under a variety of delivery patterns for primary care.

In the free enterprise systems, individual medical practice in private offices is the predominant mode of furnishing primary as well as other aspects of ambulatory service. The same applies to dental care, to eye refractions by optometrists, and even sometimes to specialized services such as physiotherapy or psychotherapy. In years past, the individual doctor often operated his office within his home, and this practice still prevails in some rural areas. As private medical practice has become more complex and also more lucrative, offices have typically been separated from homes. They are now usually found in commercial structures, sometimes in medical arts buildings catering exclusively to private doctors, dentists, pharmacists, and other health-related personnel.

Part of the doctor-patient relationship in the free enterprise setting has been the patient's payment of a fee. The amount of the fee is intended to reflect the value of the service, and the value is largely determined by the skill and time required to render it. The skill, in turn, is dependent on the years of training and experience necessary to acquire it. There are, of course, other factors in the medical market involved in the determination of fee levels—supply and demand, the general price level (inflation or deflation), the special features of a particular case, the patient's affluence, professional custom in the community, and so on. Sometimes the fees for different services are stipulated in a fee schedule that is agreed on by the professional association in a city or district. (This sort of trade agreement is designed to restrict competitive fee reductions which, it is argued, might compromise the quality of medical care, although it has been attacked recently as monopolistic in effect.) The fee paid to the doctor is intended to cover all the overhead expenses of his practice (auxiliary staff, rental, equipment, etc.) as well as his net earnings.

So firmly imbedded in the free enterprise system is this fee-for-service scheme of medical remuneration that it is generally used even when the payment for care has been collectivized through a third-party voluntary or government agency. Thus, private insurance, social insurance, and revenue-supported public medical care programs will usually pay doctors, dentists, and others on a fee basis for rendering services to designated persons. Sometimes the fees may be fixed in a negotiated fee schedule and sometimes they may be flexible, depending on the circumstances of the case. The latter policy applies in the United States social insurance Medicare program, where "usual and customary" fees (usual for the specific doctor and customary for the local area) may be charged. Under commercial insurance programs for health care, following indemnity principles, fees may be completely flexible. The insurance carrier indemnifies the patient only for a designated amount, but the practitioner may charge whatever he likes. In the so-called "service plans," sponsored by Blue Shield or Blue Cross agencies in the United States (and similar bodies in Australia), providers of service have ordinarily agreed with the agency to charge only the designated fee, extra billings being allowed for exceptionally difficult cases or for persons of high income. The effects of the fee-for-service and other methods of paying health care providers on their performance will be explored later.

In the free enterprise setting a century ago, primary health care was provided mainly by family doctors or general practitioners. As medical science has become more complex, especially since 1900, an enlarging proportion of doctors have entered specialties and an increasing share of services have been rendered by specialists. Certain specialists continue to give primary care, as well as secondary-level service for more complex conditions. Thus, pediatricians in the United States and Canada render much of the primary care to children, especially in well-to-do families, as well as more complex services. The same applies to internists (specialists in internal medicine) who treat many adults of both sexes, and to obstetrician-gynecologists for adult women. As the proportion of general practitioners has declined, this sort of adjustment to meet the needs for primary health care has been inevitable. (This is not so true in the welfare state countries where general practitioners are more numerous.)

Another adjustment to the specialization trend in the free enterprise setting has been private group medical practice. A team of medical and surgical specialists working together can compensate for the narrowness (with greater depth, of course) of each doctor and achieve a comprehensive range of competence. For the first half century or so after its beginnings by the Mayo brothers in 1885, American group practice was nearly always of a multispecialty composition.

Since the 1930s, groups of specialists in one field have also been frequently formed to achieve round-the-clock and seven-day-a-week coverage more conveniently. By the 1970s, over 20 percent of clinically practicing physicians in the United States were engaged in some form of group practice, and the proportion continues to grow. Many group practices include general practitioners as well as dentists and an increasingly wide range of allied health personnel (see Chapter 3). The vast majority of group practices derive their incomes from fee payments, whether from individuals or third-party agencies, although the doctors may be paid in a variety of ways. A common method is by salary (which varies with qualifications, seniority, etc.) plus a portion of the fees derived from the particular doctor's work.

Aside from group practice, primary care and other components of ambulatory service have become subject to organization in numerous other ways within the free enterprise setting. As subsystems for special populations or certain diseases, clinic programs have been established for the indigent, for industrial workers, for school children, for the mentally ill, for military personnel, for venereal disease, for emergency patients coming to hospitals, and along many other lines. Doctors serving in these clinics are most often paid by part-time salaries (that is, at a fixed rate per hour), and in aggregate these organized patterns of health care delivery may constitute a substantial fraction of ambulatory service, perhaps as much as 50 percent nationally. The predominant single pattern of primary care delivery in the United States, however, remains the individual doctor in a private office.

The welfare state systems of Western Europe, Japan, New Zealand, and Australia also retain as their predominant pattern of primary health care delivery the private medical or dental practitioner. By adopting the fee-for-service as the main method of remuneration, these systems have in some ways even crystallized this delivery model. Nevertheless, social insurance programs have also created pressures for modifying delivery patterns, if only in the interests of economy with monies that become publicly very visible.

Most of the changes induced by social insurance have been in the hospital-based sector of medical care, where the costs are much greater than those for ambulatory care. These specialized services will be discussed on page 121. Even for primary health care, however, certain mutual sickness funds in Germany organized dispensaries with salaried full-time doctors fifty years ago. More recently in France, the social security system has promoted the establishment of health centers for general practitioners where insured persons can be sure that official fee schedules will be respected. In the British National Health Service, as noted earlier, general practitioners are paid by monthly capitation amounts rather than by fee-for-service; this method can have many impacts on the doctor's medical performance, as we will see later. The British NHS has also offered direct financial inducements to the grouping of general practitioners, whether or not they

occupy one of the hundreds of health centers built by the local authorities.
More than half of British general practitioners are now working in teams of two
or more, a pattern that was rare before social insurance.

The Scandinavian setting, with its large rural areas, has generated another
delivery pattern for primary care. "District doctors" are appointed in Norway
and Sweden to serve the general medical needs of total populations. For certain
preventive services (e.g., examinations of school children) they are paid a government salary and given the assistance of nurses, but most of their incomes is
derived from fees paid by the social insurance program. As government employees, the district doctors typically work in facilities furnished by the local
community, and they have many sociomedical obligations unknown in ordinary
private practice.

Because of the strong linkage of specialists to hospitals in most of the welfare state systems, the great majority of community doctors are general practitioners who lack any hospital appointment. Although this may deprive them of
the stimulating effect of a hospital environment, it strenghthens the role of primary care. In welfare states such as Canada, Norway, Belgium, and Great Britain,
one does not see the fervent drive to train nurse practitioners or physician assistants to replace the doctor as the provider of much primary health care. Instead,
the general practitioner, who remains in much higher proportions, is being
strengthened with continuing education, more support personnel, health center
quarters, and in other ways. The British GP capitation payment method, moreover, links over 98 percent of the population to a particular primary doctor at
all times, and he provides general surveillance and coordination of services for
all the patients on his list—a helpful and protective role that is often sorely lacking in the bewildering American medical care scene.

Regarding personal patient-doctor relationships, it may be noted that in
Western Europe they are as close, or perhaps closer, than in the United States.
With small or no fees to pay regardless of personal wealth, the European patient
tends to have a stable and warm relationship with his primary care doctor. Opinion polls in Europe invariable show an overwhelmingly high level of satisfaction
with the medical care systems, in contrast to the findings of such surveys in
America. Competition among doctors still operates and furnishes incentives
for each physician to satisfy the needs of his patients. A very much lower rate
of malpractice lawsuits in Western Europe and Canada than in the United States
may well reflect, in part, fewer hostile patients who are angry when poor medical
results still entail substantial fees.

In transitional countries, the patterns of delivery of primary health care
are numerous. They vary generally with the social class of the patient. Isolated,
largely Indian, mountain or jungle populations in Latin America still rely mainly
on local traditional healers. In the larger towns of rural regions, health centers
and outpatient departments of hospitals operated by ministries of health are

more frequently used. In such facilities the patient is served by salaried doctors, nurses, and other trained auxiliary personnel. In the main cities of each province and the national capital, charitable hospitals are also available. The outpatient services in these hospitals tend to be of meagre quality, but quantitatively the resources are more plentiful. Regularly employed workers have the advantage of access to services at social security polyclinics; the medical and associated staffs in these are found in larger numbers and receive higher salaries than those under ministry or charitable agencies, and the quality of services is probably correspondingly better. For the affluent upper-middle-class or elite families in the cities, attendance by private doctors is the general rule. Even for primary care, the affluent families will have their children seen by specialized pediatricians, while adults consult internists or obstetrician-gynecologists. When lower-middle-class families visit a private doctor, he is more likely to be a general practitioner.

In the acknowledged underdeveloped countries, the traditional village healers are the principal resource for primary care. Although they lack scientific training, they know the people and understand their problems; insofar as most, if not all, diseases have some psychosomatic aspects, these healers can doubtless be helpful. Many illnesses are self-limiting, and the patient will recover regardless of the treatment. If he does not, he may then decide to seek help from a governmental health center or hospital. In small villages, the local healer is likely to be a farmer who treats the sick part of his time; in larger settlements, he may work on a full-time basis. Childbirth is ordinarily assisted by a midwife, typically an older village woman who has had several children of her own. Both healer and midwife may be paid for their services by money or by barter.

In the larger towns or cities of the underdeveloped countries, there are greater resources for modern medical care. There are health centers staffed with trained medical assistants and nurses, and there are hospitals with doctors. Government funds are so limited, however, that, unlike the policy in the transitional countries, patients are often charged small fees to support these public services (and also, it is claimed, to enhance the patient's appreciation of their value). Most of the physicians serving on salaries in urban public facilities also have private medical practices, and an occasional doctor, trained abroad, may be engaged entirely in private practice. The handful of wealthy families consult these private doctors for all their medical care, and some lower-middle-class people will seek private care for especially disturbing illnesses.

In the socialist countries, developed on the Soviet model, primary health care is ordinarily obtained at the government health center or polyclinic nearest to the patient's home. For each 2,000 adults in the Soviet system, there is a therapeutist or general practitioner; this doctor is expected to provide primary treatment and preventive services for all the adults in a defined geographic district. If a patient does not like the doctor covering his area, he may choose another one at the same or another health center. Such a step, however, is said to be taken only rarely. When a specialist is required, the patient is referred to him in the same polyclinic or at a nearby hospital. All Soviet doctors work only six to seven hours a day, including the time allotted for home visits. It is expected that each general practitioner should spend a half hour daily in health education work.

Special emphasis is given in the socialist systems to the care of children, and in the USSR a pediatrician is responsible for each 1,000 children in a defined area. The Soviet pediatrician, however, is not regarded as a specialist in the American sense but rather as a general practitioner for children. Medical education has three principal tracks after the first two years: general medicine, pediatrics, and hygiene. Thus, by the end of the six-year curriculum (the standard length, after secondary school, in all European countries), those who have chosen the pediatric path are already focused in this field. Although the majority of all Soviet doctors are women, the proportion of women in pediatrics is about 90 percent. Almost every ambulatory care facility has pediatricians for the children as it has therapeutists for the adults. In the cities, there may even be entire polyclinics, with a full range of specialists, devoted entirely to children. The same primary care doctor sees the child when he is sick and for periodic examinations when he is well.

Another priority group in the Soviet system are industrial workers. At larger factories or mines, there are fully staffed clinics where workers may be seen for any condition, not solely for job-related injuries or diseases. Some workers may use the industrial clinic as their main source of primary care, whereas others use their neighborhood unit. In recent years, more emphasis has been put on the community facilities, and industrial clinics have become somewhat more specialized in work-related disorders. They are not constrained by any competitive considerations, however, from treating nonoccupational conditions.

In most health centers and polyclinics where primary care is given, *feldshers* and nurses are on the staff to assist the doctor. Very thinly settled rural areas in the Soviet Union are served by small health stations staffed only by *feldshers* or *feldsher*-midwives. These personnel are supervised by a doctor at the nearest health center, but they are trained to handle common ailments themselves and to recognize cases requiring referral.

Finally, we should note the special arrangements for primary care for the huge population of the People's Republic of China. The concept of the "barefoot doctor" and his or her training and functions were discussed earlier. This part-time primary health care worker is employed in a production brigade and paid by the commune for his work according to a point system similar to that used to compensate agricultural workers. Since the commune is equivalent to a unit of local government, which all the members support, no charges are made for the services. Only if the patient must be referred to a health center or hospital is he expected to pay a small fee; if the commune has a health cooperative, it pays the fee for him. The barefoot doctor, one must realize, uses ancient herbal remedies and acupuncture, as well as modern scientific techniques. In addition, there are both Western-style and traditional Chinese doctors offering primary care at health centers in communes and also in larger cities. The Maoist strategy of combining modern and traditional medicine has meant that the traditional healer learns about modern Western medicine and vice versa. The patient makes the choice of which type of doctor he wishes to consult.

Specialties and Hospitalization

The increasing complexities of medical science have led to specialization of functions everywhere, but the patterns of delivery of specialized services differ among countries. In ancient Egypt, there were artisans who specialized in the treatment of different types of ailment, but later, from the time of Hippocrates in Greece, the doctor was ideally a generalist. After the rise of university education in the Renaissance, this broad role was embodied in trained physicians except for surgeons who were regarded as needing only lowly manual skills. Not until the early nineteenth century was surgery fully reintegrated into medicine. Specialization then principally took the form of separate occupations: pharmacy, dentistry, midwifery, nursing, and so on.

In the late nineteenth and early twentieth centuries, specialization began to develop within the medical profession. With the spectacular pace of scientific advances, rapid urbanization, and the rising level of public education, after about 1920 the specialties in medicine grew rapidly. This was especially marked in the wealthy industrialized nations but occurred to some extent everywhere. In most countries, specialization was linked to hospitals, where large numbers of patients with certain diagnoses were concentrated. The hospitals of North America were exceptional in inviting almost every doctor to bring his seriously ill patients into hospitals. Similarly, out-of-hospital or community medical practice became the province of specialists as well as of general practitioners. This background accounts for much of the difference seen today in the characteristics of the medical specialties in various countries.

In the United States setting—freewheeling and laissez faire—specialization developed more rapidly than anywhere else, and there has always been both a technical and an economic significance to the specialties. Not only did expanding knowledge lead to the subdivision of practice into many disciplines, but the expanding economy was able to support the higher costs of the longer training required for specialization. Because of these greater costs, along with the market dynamics of supply and demand, the fees for specialist service are higher. Larger incomes naturally attract more and more young doctors into the specialties.

Thus, as noted earlier, the proportion of specialists to general practitioners in the United States rose from about 20 percent in 1920 to about 80 percent in 1970. Not all these were certified by the various specialty boards, but they confined their work substantially to some special sector of medicine. The conspicuous lack in the 1970s was of physicians for general primary care—a problem met by establishing a specialty of family practice, by introducing family medicine into medical education, by training nurse practitioners as doctor substitutes for handling common ailments, and in other ways.

Entry into the specialties in the United States has been essentially free and unplanned. The preparation is through training in hospital residency programs, that is, working with hospital patients under the supervision of other recognized specialists for three or more years. The decision as to which specialty a young doctor would prepare for has been largely his own. Since the incomes and prestige of surgeons, for example, are high, the applicants for surgical residencies have been numerous. In response, many hospitals, both university affiliated and others, have developed such residency programs. The American Medical Association, although nongovernmental, has established a review procedure to determine whether the professional staffing and training content of these programs are adequate. If standards are met, there is no limitation put on training places in relation to the national needs for surgeons or any other type of specialist. Similarly, subspecialty training programs have developed in such fields as orthopedic or thoracic surgery, cardiology, and gastroenterology.

As a result of these highly permissive policies, the United States has a higher percentage of specialists and a lower percentage of general practitioners than any other country. There are twice as many surgeons as in Great Britain for example. It has also been found that approximately twice as high a rate of elective surgery is performed in the United States as in Britain—a fact that surely bears some relationship to the manpower supply and to the policy of having surgeons (with fee-for-service remuneration) make the decisions on surgical intervention. Numerous studies have, indeed, shown that much of the surgery done in American hospitals cannot be medically justified. At the same time, there is widespread recognition of shortages in other specialized fields, such as pediatrics and psychiatry.

In the welfare state countries of Western Europe, specialization is also highly developed but not to the level of the United States. About 50 to 60 percent of European doctors are specialists, compared with 80 percent in the United States. The difference is probably explained in large part by the much closer linkage of European specialists to hospitals and the more restrictive policies of institutional staffing. In the Scandinavian countries and Great Britain, the distinction is clear-cut; virtually all medical work in hospitals is done by full-time or nearly full-time salaried specialists. There is stiff competition for these appointments, and only the requisite numbers of doctors in each specialty are selected. Even in France, Germany, and other continental countries, where salaried hospital doctors are not universal (although they serve patients in over half the hospital beds), the medical staffs of hospitals are still relatively "closed." Only highly qualified specialists, whether in private practice or salaried employees, are appointed.

Under these arrangement, the numbers of doctors seeking specialty status are bound to be fewer. A specialist could hardly expect to make a living without a hospital appointment, and the number of such appointments is small. With fewer applicants for specialty training, there are naturally fewer training programs. No Western European country has done completely systematic planning; in fact, every year there are young surgeons or other specialists who have completed their training and yet are not chosen for a hospital position. As a result, they are obliged to enter general practice or to leave the country. To avoid such wasted efforts and frustration, many welfare state countries are limiting their specialty training programs in accordance with the objective national needs. Canada has also embarked on a major specialty planning effort along these lines.

In both the transitional and the underdeveloped countries, the proportions of specialists are much lower than in the developed countries. Opportunities for specialty training are relatively limited, and the young doctors who wish to specialize must often go abroad for further study. Numerous hospital training positions in the United States and Europe are, in fact, occupied by foreign doctors from the less developed countries. Specialists in Africa, Asia, and Latin America are nearly all confined to the main cities where they typically work both in hospitals on part-time salaries and in private practice. Only the small number of hospital patients who are private yield individual fees, and the rate of elective surgical procedures is relatively low.

In the socialist countries, also, specialization has grown but less than in the welfare state countries. Deliberate emphasis has been put on an abundant supply of primary care doctors to meet the commonplace needs of adults and children. Hospitals are staffed solely with salaried specialists but, since they are all full-time, their ratios per 100 beds are lower than in Western Europe and much smaller than in the United States. The numbers of specialists trained in each field are calculated in relation to the hospital posts to be filled. With this policy, competition occurs at an early stage for training opportunities, rather than later for hospital staff appointments.

Although private specialty practice for ambulatory patients is almost unknown in the socialist countries, there are many specialists in the public polyclinics and hospital outpatient departments. These positions tend to go to the more junior specialists, with the more senior personnel, aside from young doctors in training, holding the hospital posts. In Cuba, where the over-all supply of specialists is not yet high enough, hospital specialists may also have to spend some time in the polyclinics. In the USSR, there is a deliberate rotational policy between hospital and polyclinic specialists, so that each can learn to appreciate the problems of the other.

With the generally close ties of specialists to hospitals in almost all countries except the United States and Canada and to a lesser extent Australia and Japan, the medical staff organization in the hospitals of most countries is rather structured. The chief of each clinical department has a great deal of control over the methods of case management in his jurisdiction. Many patients may be treated by young doctors in training, but their work is quite closely supervised. In the larger hospitals, there are systematic ward rounds at which the younger doctors report to the senior staff and all cases are discussed.

In these structured settings, there is much less need for the peer review procedures that have developed in American and Canadian hospitals, somewhat in compensation for the autonomy of the private practitioner. Tissue committees, medical audits, record review procedures, and so on that are required for accreditation of American hospitals are seldom found in the more structured settings. Medical staff discipline is built into the day-to-day activities of the doctors. There are exceptions, of course, as in Belgium where the individual specialist's autonomy is closely guarded once he has made the grade of getting a hospital staff appointment. In most public hospitals of Western Europe, however, the right of patients to complain to official authorities if they are dissatisfied is the safeguard for the quality of medical performance. A physician found by his colleagues to be doing poor work, moreover, can be subjected to greater supervision or, as a last resort, removed from the hospital staff.

In the centrally controlled government hospital networks of both transitional and underdeveloped countries, supervision is applied throughout the system as a whole. Higher authorities of the ministry of health or the social security body inspect hospitals periodically and make judgments on the quality of both professional and institutional performance. The reliability of this sort of supervision is naturally variable, depending on the competence and integrity of the top officials. Quality supervision on a system basis is exercised similarly in the socialist countries. The watchdog to protect the patient's interest is generally the local political party organization. In Poland, there are periodic inspections by representatives of the regional academy in each medical specialty; a critical judgment by these external examiners can result in sending an individual doctor to a center for further training or some other disciplinary actions.

Specialization everywhere in the world seems to have led to a certain dehumanization of doctor-patient relationships. The specialist inevitably focuses his attention on a diseased organ or some other narrow aspect of the patient rather than the person as a whole. This may, indeed, mean very skillful performance within the specialized sector; we know that modern surgery and other therapies have saved many lives that would once have been lost. However, this mechanization of much patient care has led to demands for greater medical humanism and sensitivity in countries of every type. It is a factor in the swing of the specialty pendulum in recent years toward greater emphasis on general practice and family medicine.

At the same time, there has been a growing realization, especially in the European welfare states, that the general medical practitioner can fall behind the times in medical technology. He may become strong on interpersonal relations and weak on diagnostic and therapeutic science. To cope with this, many countries are developing stronger programs of continuing education for general practitioners. Various financial and prestigious awards are offered as incentives to encourage such studies regularly. Efforts are also being made to break down the barriers between community practice and hospitals, not by forming departments of general practice in hospitals, as in the United States, but by inviting the GP to work in a hospital outpatient department, to attend clinical conferences, and to make direct use of the hospital's diagnostic resources for his office patients. In a sense, these efforts are approaching a compromise pattern between the closed-staff policies of European hospitals and the open-staff policies of American hospitals. The position of the general practitioner under social insurance programs is also being strengthened by alteration of fee schedules to upgrade the payments for GP care.

Payment Methods and Medical Performance

The performance of doctors and other health personnel is inevitably influenced by the methods by which they are paid. As already discussed, the fee-for-service pattern predominates in the free enterprise countries for all medical care, and for most out-of-hospital care in the welfare states as well. A salary or payment on a time basis is the general rule for all services in the socialist countries, inside hospitals in many welfare states, and in several organized subsystems of the developing countries of both types. The implications of these and other methods of remuneration for the quantity and quality of patient care should be explored further.

The fee system developed with the decline of feudalism and settlement of doctors in the cities as independent tradesmen. They competed with apothecaries and with various artisans who claimed to have skills in treating certain ailments. The early medical societies were designed to advance the stature of physicians as against other healers and also to control competition among themselves. These objectives were implemented with codes of medical ethics and schedules of medical fees to be followed in a region or a nation.

With industrialization, when first voluntary and then mandatory, health insurance programs arose in Europe, the fee system was well established. It was natural that the insurance mechanism should simply be applied to the payment of medical fees. In Germany and other parts of Central Europe, where health insurance first arose, the responsibility for paying fees was transferred from individuals to pooled sickness funds. By the time the later programs of social insurance evolved in the Scandinavian countries and then in France, doctors had come to regard this arrangement as infringing on their independence and their personal relationships with patients. Therefore, they insisted on direct cash payment by the patient, who would later seek reimbursement from the insurance fund. In this way, the doctor was not obligated to make any contract with a third party—the insurance society or government.

Furthermore, because insurance was believed to generate excessive demand for medical care, this indemnification mechanism had another advantage in the doctors' eyes. When the insurance reimbursement was made at a rate less than the full cost—such as 75 to 80 percent—the patient was obliged to pay a share. This cost sharing, it was believed, would inhibit excessive utilization. Second, it was thought it would foster a better patient-doctor relationship since the patient would better appreciate a service he had paid for, in part, personally. Third, cost sharing would reduce the drain on the insurance funds. As a result of this reasoning, most of the Western European health insurance programs that developed after the 1900s (as well as those in Japan in 1921, New Zealand in 1939, Australia in 1952, and most recently in the United States) have included some degree of cost sharing or co-payment by the patient.

The fee system, with or without cost sharing, had the advantage of offering the doctor incentives for diligent work and for maximizing his services to the patient. The more services he rendered, the more he would be paid. The possibility of overservicing by the doctor was not recognized as an issue until the early twentieth century. In the pioneer German setting, the *Krankenkassen* could bargain with individual doctors for lower fees, could engage some on capitation agreements or even salaries, and could prorate (pay less than 100 percent) the fees due, in accordance with the money available each month. In 1900, the German doctors reacted by organizing the *Hartmannbund,* a kind of collective bargaining body that eventually became the economic division of the German Medical Association. In time, German physicians achieved a much greater measure of control by getting the law changed so that the sickness funds made their payments to the association of doctors rather than to individual practitioners. These payments were at rates that were collectively negotiated. Then the medical association would pay the doctors. In this way, the association could discipline individual members who were deemed to be overservicing (and thereby reducing the money available to other doctors), while also being in a position to bargain for higher payments from the insurance societies.

In Great Britain, which enacted its social insurance for general practitioner care in 1911, another approach to overservicing by the doctor or overutilization by the patient was taken. After starting on a basis that allowed the doctors in each community to use their preferred pattern of remuneration—fees, salaries, or capitation—the British Medical Association took a vote of its members. The majority decided in favor of payment according to the number of persons choosing to be on each doctor's panel. This capitation scheme was considered fairest because it would reward individual practitioners in proportion to their ability to attract patients, and yet it would not pay additionally for a higher volume of service that might be excessive. Theoretically, it would induce the doctor to maximize preventive service, since this would not only keep his patient healthy but would save him work later. It would assure the doctor a steady income in accordance with the size of his panel, moderate the day-to-day competition, reduce shopping around for doctors by patients, and minimize paper work. After the National Health Service was established in 1948 and also with the reduction of preventable infectious diseases, it was found that the pure capitation pattern did not achieve these purposes so well. It became supplemented by various special payments—fees for immunizations, higher capitation amounts for aged patients with more chronic illness, supplements for group practice or office assistants, and so on.

The cost-sharing requirement for the patient, however, was the commonest method employed to constrain medical care utilization and to control costs in the welfare state systems. It was not appreciated until much later, around 1940, that the doctor rather than the patient made the decisions that accounted for the greatest share of medical costs—the prescribed drugs, the diagnostic tests, hospitalization, the surgical procedures, and so on. It also has now become evident that co-payments have a differentially greater inhibiting effect on the use of medical care by low-income people, having little if any impact on the affluent, and perhaps discouraging the poor from seeing doctors when they should. Delays in seeking care by the poor may lead to progression of disease, the subsequent need for hospitalization, and higher costs in the end. Many European systems cope with the latter problem by exempting pensioners and other low-income persons from co-payment obligations. In any event, the whole question of cost sharing as a form of control on health insurance expenditures has become subject to increasing controversy.

In the transitional and underdeveloped countries, issues concerning methods of paying the doctor are much less prominent. With a very small market of patients who can pay any private fees, the predominant pattern of remuneration in all organized programs is the straight salary, full-time or part-time. Salaries are, of course, not all the same but depend usually on the individual's background of training, his skills, his seniority, and his responsibilities. Incentives to diligent work are furnished not by multiplication of fees or attraction of patients but by the disciplinary controls within an organization. Supervision and winning the respect of medical peers become the crucial influences. These dynamics are not always effective, and mediocrity, favoritism, or even corruption can infiltrate any organization. The same unfortunately applies to the fee pattern, and one can cite illustrations of high and low quality medical practice under both patterns. If the top leadership, however, has integrity and competence, as in

organizations such as the Mayo Clinic in the United States or the university
teaching hospitals in most countries, the salary pattern in a structured setting
lends itself to more effective quality controls than any other payment method.

The distinction between full-time and part-time salaries in the developing
countries, and to some extent also in the free enterprise and welfare states, is
important. The full-time salary can lead to a sense of loyalty and commitment
to the organization and its objectives. Its use in the Indian Medical Service and
many of the post-colonial African health care systems is designed for this purpose. By contrast, the doctor receiving a part-time salary, with several hours
each day or week devoted to private practice, has mixed loyalties. Not only is
he less likely to put his mind and heart fully unto the organized program, but
he may even obstruct attainment of its goals for his personal advantage. Thus,
it is unfortunately common for a part-time doctor to exploit his position in a
health center or clinic as a means of building up a clientele of private patients.
Seeing a clinic patient of moderate income, he may say, "For really good attention, come later to my private office." This sort of deviance is all too common
in the organized health programs of Latin America, which commonly engage
part-time salaried doctors. It is further aggravated by crowded conditions in
some public clinics, which greatly reduce the time available per patient. Unless
professional discipline is effective, the part-time doctor may even cut corners on
his allotted clinic time and give even more perfunctory care than necessary.

In the socialist countries, the full-time salary is the usual method of paying
the doctor, along with all the other personnel. Some of the abuses just mentioned
may occur, but the relatively rigorous discipline in the entire political structure of
these countries make such occurrences rare. Moreover, the emphasis on an abundant supply of doctors who are paid relatively moderate salaries means that the
time available per patient in the polyclinics or health centers is greater than in
the developing countries. As a result, there is less of the dissatisfaction that leads
South American patients to turn to private doctors and, hence, build up the
whole private sector. The vicious cycle of perfunctory public medical service,
dissatisfaction, resort to private care, enlargement of the private sector, and then
further diminution of doctor hours in the public system can be broken only by
enlarging the health manpower supply in the public sector. This has, indeed,
been the strategy of the socialist countries.

Regardless of the method of paying the doctor, medical earnings in all five
systems of health care are high relative to the incomes of other occupational
groups. Although exact data on this point are difficult to get, one can safely
say that everywhere in the world, physicians' earnings put them in the highest
10 percent of a nation's population. In free enterprise America and in the generally impoverished developing countries of both types, physicians are probably
in the highest one or two percent on the income ladder. In the welfare states,
where constraints from the social insurance systems have increased, their place

may drop to the third or fourth percentile out of 100. In the socialist countries, where positions in industrial production, teaching, and research have higher priority, physicians' relative position probably declines to between the fifth and tenth percentile. But everywhere generally the years of training required for medical qualification and the high value put on health service place the doctor in a high-income bracket.

The same cannot be said for other types of health personnel. The largest group, nurses, have suffered from two handicaps: the charitable tradition that they are working for a sacred purpose rather than material rewards, and the generally weaker economic position of women in most societies. Both of these handicaps have been reduced in recent years as nurses—especially under social insurance and other organized support systems—have recognized their bargaining potential and mobilized their strength through collective action. Sometimes this has been done explicitly through nursing labor unions and sometimes through economic committees of professional associations. Even when only a fraction of hospitals have had to negotiate with nursing unions, competition for nursing employees tends to compel the other hospitals to pay equivalent salaries. The same sort of process has led to elevation of salaries or wages for technicians, nutritionists, and other types of health personnel employed in hospitals and other organizations. Private practitioners in health fields such as pharmacy, dentistry, or optometry also earn generally lower incomes than physicians because of the supply-and-demand dynamics affecting the social value placed on their services.

In all health fields, including medicine, there seems to be a world-wide trend toward greater use of salaried remuneration owing to the general growth of organized settings for the delivery of health care, quite obvious for hospital service but true also less conspicuously for ambulatory service. This whole process is self-evident in the socialist countries, the number of which is growing. It is prominent in nearly all the developing countries; perhaps there are exceptions in the Philippines and in the Republic of (South) Korea, where government policies have deliberately maximized private health service. In the welfare states, organized health care delivery with salaried personnel has generally expanded as a reaction to the mounting costs of individual private delivery of services. Even in the United States, the proportion of doctors working on salaries has steadily risen, along with the expansion of hospitals (and their greater numbers of young doctors-in-training, outpatient or emergency physicians, etc.), the expansion of group practice, and the expansion of numerous social programs for the poor, for mental illness, and other categories.

Rural Health Care Delivery

An aspect of health care delivery on which nearly all countries have taken special steps is the provision of services to rural populations. Rural life almost everywhere has been less attractive than the cities to doctors and other personnel, re-gardless of the prevailing health care system. Moreover, insofar as medical care is provided under an unfettered free economic market, medical earnings are in-variably less in the rural areas where family incomes are lower and the demands for service less than in the cities. Thus, the disparity between rural and urban availability of health care resources is bound to be greatest where differences in living conditions and earning potentials are largest, a situation found in its most extreme degree in underdeveloped countries. The problem exists, however, in countries of every level of economic development and every political ideology.

In the affluent United States, the rural health manpower shortage has been tackled by a variety of both direct and indirect strategies. Direct actions have been taken by rural communities offering rent-free offices and a guaranteed basic salary (for certain limited public health duties) to attract doctors. Several states in the United States have offered fellowships to medical students who are then obligated to serve an equivalent number of years in a rural location needing doctors. Since 1971 the federal government has assigned young doctors, dentists, and others to rural communities through the National Health Service Corps in place of military duty. Rural enterprises such as mining or lumbering have long offered salaried positions to doctors and other health personnel.

Indirectly, the general expansion of health manpower over the last thirty years or more should have benefited rural areas; as long as there are urban short-ages, cities will attract personnel first, but if the overall supply is large enough rural areas will get a share. The Hospital Survey and Construction Act of 1946 put priority on rural hospital construction, which was also intended to improve conditions for rural medical practice. The national Medicare and Medicaid pro-grams increased medical purchasing power for the rural aged and poor by greater increments (since they started at lower levels) than for corresponding city dwell-ers. The whole regionalization movement has been largely directed to improving the quality of health services in rural areas.

In the welfare states, similar strategies are employed along with others. Over fifty years ago, the Canadian prairie provinces had rural municipal doctor plans through which local governments paid general practitioners an annual sal-ary for providing primary care to every resident. On a much wider scale, Norway and Sweden have their salaried district doctors, described earlier. Formerly, a period of service as a district doctor was mandatory, but applicants for these interesting posts have become so numerous that compulsion is no longer neces-sary.

The British National Health Service has a policy of declaring certain areas "overdoctored" with general practitioners to be paid. The result is that new graduates must go to other areas, often rural, where they are more needed. The basic operation of any national insurance scheme in welfare state countries equalizes purchasing power for doctors, except in regions that are very thinly settled. Even for the latter, the Highlands and Islands Health Program of northern Scotland demonstrates an adjustment; it pays minimum salaries to doctors who could not expect an adequate income out of capitation allotments from patients.

Use of doctor substitutes in very thinly settled areas of large territories such as the Australian Outback or the Canadian far north is another approach. Specially trained bush nurses in Australia or outpost nurses in Canada are able to cope with the great majority of medical problems, as well as giving preventive services and referring complex cases to a distant city when necessary. Special training courses have been developed for these nurses who are typically mature women with a great deal of prior experience. They are paid by national or provincial governments.

To back up these isolated nurse stations, both Canada and Australia operate aerial services for transporting either patients or doctors. Communication is maintained by radio with designated centers and sometimes, when the nurse reports certain clinical findings, she can be radioed advice on how to handle the case. If the patient requires hospitalization, the airplane will fetch him. In Australia, a physician in the Royal Australian Flying Doctor Service, started as a private philanthropic agency but now subsidized by government, may be flown to the distant spot. With use of large, wheeled vehicles, mobile clinics are widely employed in the rural regions of many developing countries.

In all the industrialized countries, where medical associations tend to be well developed, information services are often maintained about communities with a relatively low supply of doctors. Under national health insurance systems, the new doctor may be reasonably confident that an area with few other practitioners is bound to yield a good professional income. Information may be furnished on the age of each area's local doctors, some of whom may be approaching retirement. Some countries have gone further with respect to immigrant physicians; several Canadian provinces are obligating new medical settlers to spend a designated number of years in a rural location before attaining citizenship. Just after World War II, a similar policy was employed by Sweden with respect to the numerous doctors seeking to leave Austria at the time.

In many transitional countries, the licensure of new medical graduates has been made conditional on spending time in a rural post. Mexico has required its period of rural social service since 1933. The new graduate is typically stationed in a small rural health center under the supervision of a provincial or district health officer. Several other Latin American countries apply a similar policy. The same has been done in Malaysia to recruit doctors for the health centers of the Rural Health Services Scheme. In Iran, military authority has been invoked to obtain service from new medical, nursing, dental, and related graduates in a Rural Health Service Corps.

The socialist countries, following the Soviet example, usually require all new medical and dental school graduates to spend two to three years in a rural post. After this they are free to move, but premium salaries are offered to induce them to stay. In very thinly settled areas, as noted earlier, *feldshers* or *feldsher*-midwives are stationed under the supervision of the nearest health center. The People's Republic of China has developed its impressive numbers of minimally trained barefoot doctors. To maintain a proper level of competence, these peasant personnel are given additional training for a week or two every year at a commune health center or a county hospital; doctors from the main cities go out periodically to furnish this training.

Delivery of Special Health Services

Regarding special sectors of health service, the patterns of delivery are often different from those for day-to-day medical care and require that we give them brief consideration.

Treatment of the mentally ill has demanded special strategies in every country. In an earlier section, we saw how the proportion of hospital beds devoted exclusively to mentally disturbed or retarded patients differed among countries. In general, the more economically advanced countries have a higher proportion of beds for mental cases; how much of this reflects a greater incidence of mental disorder owing to competitive pressures, urbanization, and so on, and how much a higher level of recognition of these conditions along with more resources to handle them is not clear. In any event, the mounting allocation of beds for mental disorder generated several important modifications of delivery patterns for psychiatric service in the industrialized countries.

With the advent of the tranquilizing and therapeutic drugs and the therapeutic community (sensitive care rather than forceful restriction) after World War II, mental hospitals in Great Britain and America opened their doors. With the open door replacing the locked gate and barred window, most mental hospital admissions became voluntary rather than by legal commitment. Although compulsory hospitalization continues for the dangerously disturbed patient, it is the declining practice in most of the welfare states as well as in the United States.

In tandem with the recent reduction of the number of mental hospital beds in the industrialized nations, there has been an expansion of ambulatory care mental clinics. Diverse types of unit have been organized: for children, for adults, for crisis intervention, for suicide prevention, for marital counseling, for alcoholism, for drug addiction, and so on. Group therapy for patients is provided as well as individual therapy; psychologists and social workers serve along with psychiatrists. Mental health clinics may be sponsored by government or by private agencies, often with public subsidy. Many clinics give follow-up care to patients discharged from mental hospitals, monitoring their drug therapy if necessary.

Another reaction against the huge, impersonal mental hospital in the more economically developed countries has been the admission of mental patients to general hospitals, usually for stays of under thirty days. This practice has brought psychiatrists in closer contact with other physicians, enhancing general medical sensitivity to the psychological aspects of somatic disease. In Great Britain and a few other countries, special small hospital units have developed for the care of some disturbed patients by day, sending them home at night. Others care for the patient by night, while he lives or works in the community by day. These "day" or "night" hospitals are believed to be more effective therapeutically, as well as being less expensive than traditional types.

A unique pattern for the care of mental patients has been operating for centuries in Belgium. In the old town of Gheel, several hundred mentally ill patients are cared for in the homes of townspeople who are paid by the government for this service. Starting from religious inspiration in the Middle Ages, the Gheel approach has proved to be an effective substitute for mental hospital care, but it has not been easy to replicate elsewhere. Foster homes for mentally retarded children, however, are widely used in the more developed countries.

Still another means of reducing the census of large mental hospitals has been the care of aged senile patients in various sorts of general custodial facilities, discussed on page 133. Most senile psychotic patients, it has been learned, can be well cared for without physical restraints and with a program of activity and diversion.

In both the transitional and underdeveloped countries, mental illness care has been a low priority. The large and meagerly staffed custodial institution, where the patient gets little if any therapy, is still unfortunately the general rule. Admission is virtually limited to the poor of all ages who have created disturbances in their communities and cannot be handled in a family. Mental health clinics are very weakly developed, except occasionally in a few large cities. Private psychiatrists are a luxury for the wealthy.

The socialist countries also do not devote a great share of hospital beds to psychiatric care, but those available are well staffed. Conditions now in the mental hospital near Havana present a striking contrast to conditions before the Cuban Revolution. Under the socialist, materialist philosophy, little confidence is placed in Western-style psychotherapy and much more in drugs, physical medicine, and group activities. The causes of mental illness are mainly linked to the patient's relationships with his fellow-men, and treatment is directed toward improving his social consciousness and capacities.

The general approach of a country to aging and long-term illness parallels in many ways the psychiatric field. In the more affluent nations, the proportion of the population 65 years and over has been rising steadily, and this has naturally created special problems. Along with the greater mobility and urbanization of industrialized populations goes less family stability, so that aged relatives are less likely to be kept as part of an extended family. Moreover, more people live on to old age, so that the net burden on the young for their care is proportionally greater. In persons past seventy or eighty years of age, of course, the prevalence of disabling chronic disease becomes steadily greater.

To cope with these burdens of old age and chronic illness, the more economically advanced countries have developed all sorts of institutional facilities. In the free enterprise United States, these facilities are predominantly under private commercial auspices as nursing homes or various types of private residential units. A small proportion of custodial beds are in religious or public institutions. In the welfare states, these facilities are predominantly under government auspices; some are under church or other nonprofit sponsorship, but very few are private. A rising proportion of patients in general hospitals, furthermore, are over sixty-five years of age; some hospitals have special sections for aged and long-term patients.

Regardless of institutional sponsorship, the costs of maintenance of long-term patients in the wealthier countries are usually borne by social insurance programs. Old-age pensions are used for the feeble aged who do not require strictly medical or nursing care; health insurance or public assistance funds pay, in whole or in part, for medical services to the aged. The United States legislation on Medicare for the aged is unique in the world, with its confinement of social insurance health care benefits to the aged and the totally disabled, while the rest of the population is expected to be covered by voluntary health insurance. In the United States and in all the welfare state countries, there are also social insurance cash benefit programs for permanent disability or invalidity that help to pay for the medical and custodial care of severely disabled persons.

To reduce the occupancy of general hospital beds by long-term patients, organized home care programs have been launched in many larger cities of the affluent countries. Sometimes these programs are sponsored by general hospitals, but more often they are the responsibility of visiting nurse associations or public welfare agencies. By having nurses visit the patient at home, assist with various medical procedures, educate the family about proper patient care, and so on, many chronic patients can be kept out of expensive hospital beds. It depends, of course, on the availability of an intact family. In Canada and Western Europe, visiting nurses are sometimes attached to residential buildings for old people to help them with the intercurrent illness that so often occurs.

Rehabilitation programs in the wealthier countries have also developed to help severely disabled people recover the ability to function independently and, possibly, to work. In addition to medical care, these programs usually include prolonged training in all sorts of activities of daily living, education for new types of employment, job placement, and much psychosocial support. Such programs may occasionally exist for disabled soldiers in even the developing countries, but for the general civilian population they are rare in Latin America, Asia, and Africa. In the affluent countries, there are also numerous general activity programs for senior citizens to prevent senile deterioration. These programs are usually organized around various sorts of community social centers under governmental or sometimes religious sponsorship.

Special programs for the aged and chronically sick are seldom found in the transitional countries and almost never in the underdeveloped countries. Occasionally, a charitable *beneficencia* society in Latin America may operate a facility for the aged, but its capacity is usually much smaller than the need and its resources are typically meager. In the scale of priorities of the developing countries, care of the aged cannot rate very high in relation to other health and welfare problems. Among the small class of affluent families in these countries, the care of an aged and feeble parent at home is the general rule, usually with the assistance of several low-paid servants.

The socialist countries protect the aged and chronically ill largely through pension systems, and only to a small extent through custodial facilities. Special homes for the aged do not occupy so important a place as in the welfare states because of different priorities and also because the extended family is usually expected to care for aged relatives. This pattern predominates in the social fabric of the USSR and the People's Republic of China where grandparents tend the small children while both parents work; then, when the grandparents become old and feeble, they are cared for in the same family home. Both the USSR and China operate custodial facilities for the disabled aged without family homes.

Special institutional care has long been available for tuberculosis and leprosy patients in all types of country. As these diseases have declined and as tuberculosis has become manageable with drugs taken at home, sanitariums have been converted to other purposes. Most frequently, they have been modified into institutions for the aged who have various chronic diseases; sometimes they have been altered to serve as general hospitals.

In more recent decades, cancer has been the subject of special programs. Throughout the United States, there are numerous hospitals specializing in the treatment of cancer patients and in research on this difficult problem, but care in these institutions is ordinarily financed privately. In Canada, several provinces previously designated cancer a "social disease," meaning that its treatment was carried out at public expense. With nation-wide hospital and physicians' care insurance in Canada, cancer costs are now met in the same way as those for any other disease. Nevertheless, Saskatchewan still supports a special Cancer Commission, which furnishes radiation therapy to any cancer patient (the world's first cobalt bomb therapy unit, incidentally, was developed here). Norway maintains a special Radium Hospital with similar purposes, and treatment in this facility is financed more heavily from general revenues than are ordinary hospitals, which are paid through social insurance.

In the transitional countries, there are often cancer hospitals operated by private societies that mainly serve patients from the upper classes. Most other cancer patients are treated in the regular general hospitals. The socialist countries also have special cancer hospitals to which any patient may be referred.

Finally, we will briefly discuss dental services. In the United States, the delivery of dental services is overwhelmingly private and given at the offices of individual dentists. Even voluntary insurance has been only weakly developed to cover the costs. Dental clinics are maintained for school children from needy families in some large cities and for pregnant women getting prenatal care from local health departments, but for the great majority of the population, dental care is a matter of purely personal responsibility.

Even in the welfare states of Western Europe, socially organized and financed dental services are largely limited to children. The major exception is Great Britain, where dental care for all age groups is a benefit of the National Health Service, although various co-payments are required for prosthetic services. Children are treated in dental clinics operated by public authorities, whereas adults visit private dental offices. The supply of dentists is less than the need, however, so that much dental disorder goes untreated.

Exceptionally well-developed dental services for children are operated in Norway and Sweden where the supply of dentists is unusually high—about 1:1200 population, compared to 1:2000 in the United States. Under government authorities, these Scandinavian countries have organized clinics where all school children may come for complete care up to eighteen years of age. It is expected that experience with this service will also have educational value, so that the habit of regular dental care will be carried into adult life, even though it must then be paid for privately. Similar public dental clinics are operated in other European countries although they are not so well staffed.

A major change in delivery patterns for dental care was launched in New Zealand in 1920. Faced with a severe shortage of dentists and evidence of massive dental neglect in military draftees, the school dental nurse program was conceived. Young women who had completed secondary school were given two years of intensive training in the examination and treatment of school children, including drilling and filling carious teeth, as well as prophylaxis. The trained dental nurses were stationed in the schools with necessary equipment and were periodically supervised by a government dentist. Eventually, all school children in New Zealand up to thirteen years of age were served by this new type of dental health worker, and the program was enormously successful and popular. The dental health of New Zealand children soon exceeded that of the children in any other country.

The New Zealand dental nurse concept, although viewed skeptically by most dentists in the United States and Europe, has now been emulated by about twenty other nations, mostly in the British Commonwealth. With variations in the equipment provided, the degree of supervision, and other details, it has been applied in England, Australia, Canada, Malaysia, Nigeria, and elsewhere. Even though these rapidly trained dental personnel may terminate their work through marriage much sooner than fully trained professional dentists, the quality of their service has been found to be good by a World Health Organization study, and the benefit-cost ratio is clearly positive. With less training, these dental personnel render a much wider range of service than the American college-trained dental hygienist who is so legally constrained in her functions. In most welfare states, however, and in the United States, dental associations have opposed this innovation, ostensibly on grounds of protecting quality standards. It seems more likely that financial considerations are involved, even though most children do not get adequate care from dentists. In time, one may predict that the dental nurse idea will gradually spread, perhaps by expanding the functions of dental hygienists, changing the role of chairside dental assistants, or in other ways. Special clinics in school buildings, moreover, have great logistic advantages.

For the great majority of the population in underdeveloped and transitional countries, restorative dental service is essentially nonexistent. Badly decayed and painful teeth in children or young adults are typically extracted (often by a doctor or medical auxiliary), as are loose teeth with periodontal deterioration in aged persons. In these countries, completely toothless old persons are relatively common.

In Australia and some European countries, the edentulous adult of low income is sometimes served by a denturist. As mentioned earlier, denturists are technical workers who take plastic mouth impressions and prepare complete upper and lower dentures without the participation or supervision of a professional dentist. Although the quality of their work is not high, they meet needs for poor people at low prices.

In the socialist countries, dental service is a benefit of the general health service system, but in relation to other needs it has not received high priority. Children are the favored group, as in the welfare states. For prosthetic work (crowns and bridges) in adults, there are often extra personal charges. The dental manpower problem has been addressed by training increasing numbers of dental doctors who are educated for a period about midway between that of the European dentist and that of the New Zealand dental nurse. Working in health centers and polyclinics, these personnel do most of the day-to-day restorative and preventive service in both children and adults. For more complex oral procedures and for general supervision of this service, there are stomatologists, who are essentially physicians specializing in disorders of the teeth and mouth.

Dental health problems on a world level are inadequately met in even the most affluent countries. The greater hope appears to lie in the prevention of dental disease, a subject to be considered in the next chapter.

Readings

Anderson, Ronald et al., *Medical Care Use in Sweden and the United States: A Comparative Analysis of Systems of Behavior,* Chicago: University of Chicago, Center for Health Administration Studies, 1970.

Benyoussef, A. and A. F. Wessen, "Utilization of Health Services in Developing Countries–Tunisia," *Social Science and Medicine, 8*:287-304 (May 1974).

Bice, Thomas W. et al., "Economic Class and Use of Physician Services," *Medical Care, 11*:287-296 (July-August 1973).

Biological Sciences Communication Project, *Delivery of Health Care in Less Developed Countries–A Literature Search,* Washington, D.C.: BSCP, June 1973.

British Office of Health Economics, *Medical Care in Developing Countries,* London: BOHE, 1972.

Brown, R. E., "Augmenting Medical Care in the Remote Areas of Developing Countries," *Clinical Pediatrics, 5*:582-584 (October 1966).

Council of Europe, *Future Organization of Medical Practice in Europe,* New York: Manhattan Publishing Co., 1972.

Dewdney, J. C. H., *Australian Health Services,* Sydney: John Wiley & Sons, 1972.

Dutt, P. R., *Rural Health Services in India: Primary Health Centres,* 2nd ed., New Delhi: Central Health Education Bureau, 1965.

Evang, Karl, *Health Services, Society, and Medicine,* London: Oxford University Press, 1960.

First International Congress of Group Medicine, *New Horizons in Health Care,* Winnipeg: Canadian Association of Medical Clinics, 1970.

Fulcher, Derrick, *Medical Care Systems: Public and Private Health Coverage in Selected Industrilised Countries,* Geneva: International Labour Office, 1974.

Gershenberg, I. and M. A. Haskell, "The Distribution of Medical Services in Uganda," *Social Science and Medicine, 6*:353-372 (June 1972).

Hopwood, B. E. C., "Provision of Medical Care in Developing Countries," *Proceedings of the Royal Society of Medicine, 63*:1196-1201 (1970).

Hughes, James P. (ed.), *Health Care for Remote Areas,* Oakland, Calif.: Kaiser Foundation International, 1972.

Institute for Health Statistics, *Czechoslovak Health Services 1965,* Prague: Ministry of Health, 1966.

Kalimo, Esko et al., "Inter-relationships in the Use of Selected Health Services: A Cross-National Study," *Medical Care, 10*95-108 (March-April 1972).

Kiev, Ari, *Psychiatry in the Communist World,* New York: Science House, 1968.

———, *Transcultural Psychiatry,* New York: Free Press, 1972.

Kilama, W. L. et al., "Health Care Delivery in Tanzania" in *Towards Ujamaa, Twenty Years of Tanu Leadership,* G. Ruhumbika (ed.), Dar Es Salaam: East African Literature Bureau, 1974.

Kohn, Robert and Kerr L. White, *Health Care: An International Study* (Report of the World Health Organization/International Collaborative Study of Medical Care Utilization), London: Oxford University Press, 1976.

MacGraith, Brian G., *Medical Aid in the Emergent World*, Greenock: University of Glasgow Press, 1970.

McWhinney, I. R., "General Practice in Canada," *International Journal of Health Services, 2*:229-237 (may 1972).

Mechanic, David, "General Medical Practice—Some Comparisons Between the Work of Primary Care Physicians in the United States and England and Wales," *Medical Care, 10*:402-420 (1972).

Medalie, J., "The Present and Future of Primary Medical Care in Israel," *International Journal of Health Services, 2*:285-296 (May 1972).

Newell, Kenneth W. (ed.), *Health By the People*, Geneva: World Health Organization, 1975.

Rabin, David L. and Patricia J. Bush, "The Use of Medicines: Historical Trends and International Comparisons," *International Journal of Health Services, 4*:61-87 (1974).

Roemer, Milton I., "Colombian Health Services in the Perspective of Latin American Patterns," *Milbank Memorial Fund Quarterly, 46*:203-212 (April 1968).

———, "General Physician Services under Eight National Patterns," *American Journal of Public Health, 60*:1893-1899 (October 1970).

———, "Organized Ambulatory Health Services in International Perspective," *International Journal of Health Services, 1*:18-27 (February 1971).

Rosner, M. M. and A. Savros, "Determinants of International Drug Consumption," *American Journal of Pharmacy, 12*:624-626 (1972).

Schicke, R. K., "The Pharmaceutical Market and Prescription Drugs in the Federal Republic of Germany: Cross-National Comparisons," *International Journal of Health Services, 3*:223-236 (1973).

Smith, A., "General Practice Present and Future in the United Kingdom and Europe," *International Journal of Health Services, 2*:255-262 (May 1972).

Solson, Anthony, "The Differential Use of Medical Resources in Developing Countries," *Journal of Health & Social Behavior, 12*:226-237 (September 1971).

Sundram, C. J., "The Delivery of Dental Services in the Asian Area of the Pacific Basis," *International Dental Journal, 23*:555-558 (December 1973).

Takulia, H. S. et al., *The Health Center Doctor in India*, Baltimore: Johns Hopkins Press, 1967.

Taylor, Carl E. et al., "Asian Medical Systems: A Symposium on the Role of Comparative Sociology in Improving Health Care," *Social Science and Medicine, 7*:307-318 (April 1973).

U.S. Department of Health, Education, & Welfare, *Rehabilitation of the Disabled in Fifty-one Countries*, Washington, D.C.: Government Printing Office, 1964.

Vayda, Eugene, "A Comparison of Surgical Rates in Canada and in England and Wales," *New England Journal of Medicine, 289*:1224-1229, 6 December 1973.

White, Kerr L. and J. H. Murnaghan, *International Comparisons of Medical Care Utilization*, Washington, D.C.: Government Printing Office, 1969.
World Health Organization, Regional Office for Europe, *Health Services in Europe*, Copenhagen: WHO, 1965.

7

DELIVERY OF PREVENTIVE SERVICES

With expanding knowledge the distinction between treatment and prevention of disease is increasingly difficult to make. Treatment of a communicable disease in one person prevents its spread to others, and early treatment of almost any disease can prevent its rate of advancement and more disabling effects. Nevertheless, for administrative and social reasons, preventive services have necessitated special organized efforts in all countries.

In the main, preventive health programs require services to the individual *before* he feels sick or while he is presumably well, as well as interventions in the environment. The full scope of preventive service is extremely wide, but we will consider only the highlights of five types of organized efforts, as they are applied in different types of nation. First we will discuss environmental control services, which encompass many ramifications in the physical and biological surroundings of man. The second subject will be the control of communicable diseases, which likewise involves diverse activities concerning many infectious diseases spread in different ways. Services to promote the health of expectant mothers, babies, and children in schools are the third type of preventive program. Fourth is the closely related promotion of birth control or family planning, which has acquired rising importance as the earth's population has increased. Finally, we will consider very briefly a number of other types of preventive health service—health education, occupational health services, and efforts at chronic disease control—activities that have developed irregularly in countries around the world.

Environmental Controls

The potentialities of preventing disease by recognizing the hazards of the environment were realized in ancient times. Hippocrates wrote of "Airs, Waters, and Places," warning of the hazards of fever (malaria) to persons living near swamps. The Greeks spoke of "miasms" rising from stagnant water, as did others for centuries before the anopheles mosquito was found to convey the malaria parasite. The contagiousness of the Black Plague in thirteenth century Europe was likewise recognized centuries before the *Bacillus pestis* was identified and measures of environmental control, such as eliminating rats, were instituted.

The range of environmental controls applied to prevent disease throughout the world is enormous. In general, they are greater and more thorough in nations that are wealthier and more urbanized. The congregation of people in cities has generally caused more serious environmental hazards and correspondingly more comprehensive measures of control.

In the strongly industrialized and free enterprise national settings, environmental sanitation has become highly developed with respect to hazards that were recognized early—those associated with water supply and excreta disposal. City dwellers in the United States usually take for granted the purity of the water from their indoor taps, whether in kitchen or bathroom, but this confidence rests on great historical accomplishments in sanitary engineering and daily surveillance. Water may be derived from rivers, wells, or other sources, but before the American urbanite drinks it, it has typically been treated, chlorinated, and tested meticulously. The process is generally more diligently carried out in the larger cities, but even in the smaller towns water safety is ensured by the vigilant supervision of public health authorities.

In the free enterprise setting, although the provision of water to dwelling units is generally a function of local government, it is not typically a "free" public service (as is education or police protection); rather, it is typically supported by payments of the property owner in proportion to the water consumed. In a small fraction of communities, water—like electricity or gas—is sold by private corporations that have been granted a franchise by local government. Whether public or private, local water systems in the United States are regulated by state public utility commissions and supervised for their hygienic quality by local public health authorities. There are nationally recommended, although not mandated, sanitary standards that are widely followed.

In very small towns or villages, public water supply systems may be operated by special districts covering many communities to attain economic viability. In some suburban areas, in hamlets of a few houses, or in country farmhouses, each individual family must ordinarily develop its own water supply from a well, or spring, or other source, with testing for purity done often on an individual basis. As the United States and other industrial nations have become more industrialized, the proportion of persons living outside the reach of a public water system has declined.

Sewerage systems to dispose of human excreta and waste water are nearly always local government systems, even in free enterprise settings. The costs of operating such systems are usually built into local property taxes or may be covered by individual sewer service charges. Public sewers are usually built under the streets, and the cost of connecting individual dwellings to them is charged to the home owner. Where a septic tank has already been constructed for a house, it may continue to be used (until it breaks down) to avoid this cost. Even in prosperous America, there are still thousands of homes, especially in the poorer areas, where pit privies are used for excreta disposal.

Garbage and other solid refuse disposal has, like sewage, also usually been assumed by local government, especially in larger cities. Suburban areas and small towns, however, may have private garbage collection companies that are paid by home owners on a fee basis. In certain communities, garbage may be used for landfill in low-lying areas and canyons or, where this is not feasible, it may be incinerated. Much emphasis is now being put on recovering resources and energy from municipal refuse.

We need not review all the elements of environmental sanitation in the free enterprise setting, except to generalize that in this basic sector of prevention, government action has probably been more fully accepted, politically and socially, than in the more personal sectors of prevention or in any aspect of medical treatment delivery. Inspection of food processing plants, abattoirs, dairies, and restaurants is a standard function of public health agencies. State or local sanitary codes have been promulgated. At the same time, the responsibility for sanitary conditions in dwellings is usually left up to property owners, although an increasing number of states and cities are developing housing codes. If disease-carrying insects or rats or other vectors are found, public agencies can compel the property owner to eliminate these hazards to community health. To do so, he must often employ private companies engaged in the vector extermination business. Such sanitizing services are seldom provided by government on private premises.

Environmental elements have often been used in the wealthiest countries as positive measures for health promotion. When iodine deficiency was found to be a cause of goiter, especially in inland areas, iodization of salt was sometimes made legally mandatory. Fluoridation of public water systems to prevent dental caries has for many reasons been subject to many more legal constraints, and in numerous cities has been a matter of public referenda. Some people view fluoridation as a contamination of natural water and as an invasion of individual rights. Therefore, despite evidence of substantial reduction of 40 to 60 percent in the incidence of caries in children drinking fluoridated water, many community votes have opposed this public health preventive measure. Water fluoridation has been adopted in most American cities by decisions of elected councils or legislatures (rather than general referenda), with enormous dental benefits and no harmful effects on any other parts of the body. Pasteurization of milk

to destroy pathogenic bacteria has long been required by law in nearly all jurisdictions, but addition of vitamin D to milk has been a matter of private initiative
by commercial milk distributors.

With greater industrialization and mechanization, many new environmental
hazards have been produced. Industrial fumes have polluted the atmosphere, just
as chemical wastes have contaminated streams, killing fish and creating toxic hazards from the consumption of seafood. The automobile, used by millions in the
affluent countries, has caused not only serious accident hazards, but its exhausts
have polluted the atmosphere, adding to the risk of serious respiratory diseases.
In reaction to these increasingly recognized hazards of modern industrial society,
national and state laws of expanding scope have been adopted for the control of
air pollution by industry, public utilities, and private automobiles. Similarly,
more strict water pollution control regulations are being enforced in the United
States with the substantial subsidy of the national government.

Radiation is another problem recognized relatively recently, especially
after the hazards of fallout from nuclear bomb testing were exposed. Alerted
by these dangers, the authorities have come to recognize the substantial risk of
excessive or improper use of diagnostic x rays and the unnecessary dangers of
fluoroscopic equipment formerly used in stores for determining the fit of shoes.

Tests on animals have revealed the potential hazards of food preservatives
and other food additives being innocently consumed. Pesticides or fungicides
used in agriculture have been indicted as hazards not only to agricultural workers
but also to those who later eat the fruits or vegetables or even the meat of animals fed on these products.

Within the last decade, there has emerged in the industrialized nations an
ecology movement in which many young people and professional conservation-
ists participate. Such movements are partly a reaction to the process of mechanization, perhaps partly a rejection of excessive emphasis on material comforts,
and a desire to return to nature. One does not see such movements to any great
extent in the developing countries where the *natural* environment is predominantly hostile to man.

In the welfare states, both water supply and sewage disposal systems are
virtually always entirely the responsibilities of local government. Indoor plumbing for both water and sewage has not had the technical development seen in the
United States, on the average, but public management of the networks of pipes
outside of houses has been taken for granted. It has been similar to the largely
governmental operation of railroads, airlines, and telephone-telegraph systems in
the welfare states. The costs are more likely to be incorporated in property
taxes than supported by charges on individual households.

Environmental inspections by government in Western Europe are directed
not only to food-processing plants, dairies, and restaurants but also to private
dwellings. Housing inspections occupy a good share of the time of public health

agencies in Great Britain, and measures to eliminate rats or other vermin are usually taken by government authorities rather than being left to private responsibility. Solid refuse disposal is nearly always a public responsibility in towns and cities of all sizes.

Official attitudes toward automobile safety illustrate the differences in approach to environmental hazards between the free enterprise and welfare state nations. In both types of country, seat belts must be provided in the manufacture of automobiles. The use of these safety devices is widely encouraged everywhere, but in many welfare state countries failure to buckle the belts is a violation of the law. A car occupant can be fined if he is detected in a moving car with unfastened seat belts. Likewise, the hazards of driving after drinking alcohol are well recognized everywhere and are the subject of educational campaigns, but in the Scandinavian countries, a driver—not in any accident but simply moving along—can be stopped and subjected to a breathing test for alcohol. If more than a low threshold quantity of alcohol is detected, he is punished by loss of his driving license for a period.

The general posture of welfare state countries is more disciplined and associated with stricter government controls than in the free enterprise setting. Education of people is not ignored, but it is backed up by mandatory requirements and official actions. Punishment of persons causing environmental hazards or even nuisances can be quite severe.

In the developing countries of both transitional and underdeveloped types, the meaning of environmental sanitation is quite different. Even in the main cities, the basic water and sewerage systems have not been so well constructed. The technical skills to treat and chlorinate water and to monitor its purity have not been so scrupulously developed, so that pollution is relatively common. Travelers not accustomed to local microorganisms are typically advised to drink bottled beverages that have been sterilized. Sometimes local government is too weak to maintain effective refuse disposal systems, and private garbage scavengers must be engaged. The World Health Organization in cooperation with international aid banks is engaged in a major program of helping the less developed countries provide public water systems in cities and small towns.

Much the greater problem in developing countries, however, is protection against environmental hazards in the rural regions, which generally contain most of the population. Outside of the principal cities, usually national and provincial capitals, water supply and sewage disposal systems are meagerly developed. A major task is still the construction of piped networks to transport clean water or liquid waste. Usually such projects depend on financial aid from the central government or international agencies, even when much construction labor is contributed locally. If local funds can be used to purchase sanitary engineering supplies, technical guidance on their installation and use must typically be obtained from higher levels. In the main, monitoring the effective operation of public sanitation systems, such as water or sewage treatment plants, reservoirs, swamp drainage projects, and so on, depends on technical services from provincial or central governments. Operating costs, however, must ordinarily be borne by the local community.

At the local level in developing countries, a major share of environmental sanitation goes to assisting rural villages or individual families in drilling wells or digging latrines. Water is so often collected from nearby streams or springs, easily and frequently polluted, that protected wells are almost always safer. A central government ministry of health will typically supply pumping equipment for wells and concrete slabs for latrine construction, with local sanitarians educating villagers about their installation. It is generally not so difficult to persuade rural people in developing countries of the value of efforts to produce a clean water supply. Safe excreta disposal methods are usually not so readily accepted by villagers whose habits for centuries have been simply to release excreta on the surface of the ground. Sanitary educational efforts to change these habits have been discouragingly slow in achieving effects.

Polluted water is responsible mostly for gastrointestinal infections; the same applies to disease organisms carried by flies from excreta to food, which is then ingested. A great problem in many developing countries is the diseases spread by mosquitoes and other vectors, whose bites infect the human bloodstream. Most prevalent on a world level is malaria, but filariasis, dengue fever, African sleeping sickness, and many other parasitic diseases are involved. Snails are vectors in schistosomiasis, rats in typhus fever and plague, many animals in brucellosis and rabies.

With respect to health care systems, the organized efforts to tackle diseases of the environment in developing countries are usually carried out through central government campaigns. The prevalence of vector-borne diseases, especially in the tropics, is usually nationwide. To be successful, the control efforts must be carried out with great thoroughness and technical competence. Swamp drainage and larvacidal programs were formerly the main approaches. Today, spraying houses with a liquid containing DDT or similar insecticide, to leave a residual film for destroying adult mosquitoes that carry malaria, is the main strategy, and it must be done meticulously. If a few infected mosquitoes survive, the spread of the disease will continue. Therefore, these campaigns are usually organized under a national plan. Even though sprayers and other health personnel may be recruited locally, the logistics of the campaign are designed centrally and directed typically from a special unit in the ministry of health.

The very centralization of these environmental control efforts, on the other hand, tends to aggravate the weakness of local public health administrative structures. These organizationally vertical campaigns are often the strategy for many preventive measures, even when an insect vector is not involved, so long as special equipment or skills are required. This applies to activities for the detection and control of tuberculosis and venereal disease and even to the educational efforts to improve nutrition or extend the use of family planning methods. With such policies, an effective local administrative structure for either preventive or curative services tends to be slow in developing.

Nevertheless, the short-run effects of these preventive environmental control campaigns in developing countries have often been successful. Over the last twenty years, for example, malaria has been substantially reduced around the world. The goal of complete eradication has not been reached, and some malariologists even question whether it is possible. In Ceylon, a reduction of malaria to nearly the vanishing point in 1965 was followed by a sudden recurrence of large numbers of cases when there was a temporary halt of DDT house-spraying and ecological conditions changed. Yet the massive threat of certain vector-borne diseases—schistosomiasis and filariasis are others—has induced *unified* national program efforts in situations where the provision of general medical care may be divided among several agencies. Thus, in Latin American countries, where social security and public health agencies are highly competitive, no question is raised about the full responsibility of a ministry of health for malaria control programs.

In socialist countries, the programs of environmental sanitation, as applied to preventive services generally, are somewhat more closely integrated with the personal health services. In the Soviet Union, linked to the hospital in each region is ordinarily a sanitary-epidemiological or "sanepid" station. A physician specializing in hygiene is usually in charge, assisted by various sanitation personnel. These sanepid workers are responsible for monitoring all water supplies, excreta disposal, restaurants, disease-vector problems, and so on in their area.

The urban-rural differentials in the hygiene of the environment are found in Eastern Europe as much as in Western Europe. Responsibilities for water supply and excreta disposal systems, however, tend to be vested in higher levels of government in the European socialist countries. Networks of pipes for water and sewage are constructed according to national five-year plans, and priorities depend on over-all national objectives for the development of industry, agriculture, and national defense. However, it appears that the conveniences of indoor plumbing have not had so high a priority in the socialist countries as the personal health services.

The centralized controls of environmental sanitation that characterize European socialism are much fewer in the People's Republic of China. Although general policies on a hygienic environemnt are issued by the central government and communicated through the Communist Party network, the implementation of programs is left largely to local municipalities or communes. In rural areas, wells or cisterns for clean water are constructed under local initiative, with perhaps some technical advice from the county (there are about 2,000 counties) level. Barefoot doctors are taught to instruct peasants about safe practices in the collection and use of night soil (human excreta) for fertilizer.

One of the environmental campaigns for disease control that well illustrates policies in China has been that for elimination of schistosomiasis. Technical information on the intermediary role of the snail in transmitting this parasitic disease was broadcast by the central Ministry of Health. The task of control through destruction of the vectors, however, was left to each commune. Instead of sending out national teams with snail-killing copper sulphate compounds, as done in most other countries, the leadership of each commune where the disease occurred was asked to mobilize the local peasants to destroy the snails by digging earth along the edges of all canals where the snails lived, and burying them. Massive manpower and motivation were applied instead of chemicals. It has been claimed that with this strategy new cases of schistosomiasis have been almost eliminated.

Communicable Disease Control

The control or elimination of certain communicable diseases depends mainly on intervention in man's environment along lines just discussed for malaria, schistosomiasis, gastrointestinal disorders, and other afflictions. But there are many other communicable diseases, the control or prevention of which requires different social actions, including systematic health services to individuals.

Best known is the deliberate protection of the individual through active immunization. On a world scale, the most frequently found type of immunization is smallpox vaccination. Despite early resistance to the discovery in 1796 by an English country doctor, Edward Jenner, that infection with cowpox (a mild disease in man) protected against smallpox, the technique spread rapidly, and it was more than a century before the virus of smallpox was identified. The principle of inoculation or immunization against infections has been applied to one disease after another since 1881, the year that Louis Pasteur (a chemist, rather than a doctor) demonstrated the effectiveness of inoculation with attenuated anthrax bacilli to protect sheep against anthrax.

In the wealthier industrialized countries, mass immunization has virtually eliminated many, if not most, acute communicable diseases. From the fight against smallpox in the early nineteenth century to measles in the 1970s, widespread application of immunization has protected large enough proportions of people (not necessarily 100 percent) to break the chain of passage of these diseases, leading to their enormous reduction.

The manner of operation and the thoroughness of immunization programs, however, vary appreciably among the different types of industrialized countries and even more so between these and the developing countries. As in the delivery of therapeutic services, whether ambulatory or hospital based, the main patterns of delivery of these personal preventive procedures depend on the over-all structure and function of the health service systems.

In the free enterprise setting, the majority of immunizations against acute communicable diseases are given in infancy by private physicians. Within the first three months of life, the infant typically has been vaccinated against small-pox, diphtheria, pertussis (whooping cough), tetanus, measles, poliomyelitis, and perhaps other acute infectious diseases. In most American families, this has been done by the pediatrician or general practitioner in his private office, and the patient pays a fee, even though the vaccines themselves are often produced by public health agencies and distributed to doctors without charge. These immunizations are typically given in the course of a routine examination of the baby when preventive counseling is also offered on infant feeding, hygienic care, and other matters.

Although the private pattern of protection against acute infections predominates in the free enterprise setting, it is not the only way. Infants in low-income families may be immunized in public clinics operated by health departments. Members of certain voluntary health insurance plans are entitled to immunizations through clinic facilities of the plan, although the most numerous commercial health insurance programs do not usually cover immunizations. Sometimes (with parental permission) immunizations are given by public school doctors or nurses to entering children who lack protection against certain diseases and hence create a risk for other children as well as themselves. The more common arrangement in school systems, however, is to require that entering children shall have been previously immunized against designated diseases and, if not, the parents are requested to go to a personal doctor or clinic for the necessary procedures.

Private medical service patterns have been so dominant in the free enterprise setting that public agencies, either health departments or schools, are usually very careful not to be competitive with private doctors, especially when a family is deemed able to afford the customary fees. The agencies fear medical profession hostility which, they believe, might jeopardize cooperation in other aspects of the public health program. In some American communities, immunizations in public clinics have been avoided even for the poor, and instead health or welfare departments offer fees to personal doctors for providing these services. The government agencies then confine their efforts to educating and urging families to take their children to private doctors for the necessary immunizations at public expense. In the 1920s and 1930s, when American public health agencies were growing stronger, there were many controversies with the medical profession about responsibility for immunizations. Even in the 1950s, when antipoliomyelities immunizations first became possible, many local medical societies opposed vehemently any public clinics for this preventive service.

There are many other aspects of communicable disease control beyond immunization. The reporting and isolating of cases and sometimes the quarantining of contacts are required by law in most countries. The diligence with which this is carried out by private physicians in the free enterprise setting is highly variable; it tends to vary with the severity of the disease (diphtheria, for example, is more carefully reported and isolated than measles), the social setting of the patient (a crowded tenement case will be more readily reported than one in an affluent separate dwelling), and the social mindedness of the doctor. Thoroughness of reporting and isolation also tend to mount when other cases have been reported and the doctors sense a possible epidemic. The notification of the health department about a communicable disease case, especially in a crowded neighborhood, may signal a visit by a public health nurse to the home to advise the family about isolation procedures.

Venereal diseases, principally gonorrhea and syphilis, are not preventable with immunization, but many other measures for their control or reduction can be carried out. Special clinics are operated by health departments for their prompt treatment and to render them noncommunicable, but in the free enterprise countries the majority of VD patients are treated by private doctors. This has been particularly true since the advent of penicillin made therapy much simpler and faster than before 1940. Public health agencies still send out nurses or VD investigators to trace contacts of patients reported by private doctors or seen at public clinics. In populations under special risk, such as young military men, VD prophylaxes may be used before sexual exposure. Sex education in the secondary schools is promoted, although this has been a subject of controversy. Prohibition of organized prostitution is the prevailing legal policy in the United States, even though nonorganized or clandestine prostitution may present equivalent hazards.

The approach to tuberculosis control in the free enterprise setting has been along many fronts. Early detection of cases through routine chest x rays has become a widespread technique. Such x rays may be taken under organized arrangements in factories, schools, general hospitals, public clinics, military settings, and so on, as well as in private medical offices. The great reduction in tuberculosis incidence and deaths began more than a century ago, well before the start of the case-detection programs, due probably to improvements in general living conditions. But the prompt detection and treatment of cases, including isolation and care of TB patients in sanitariums, has undoubtedly reduced this disease to its very low levels in the United States today.

Control of communicable diseases in the welfare state countries is generally along the lines just described for the United States, except for significant differences in the proportions of certain organized programs. Thus, immunizations of infants, although given both by private doctors and public clinics, are much more frequently done by the latter, not only because of the wider acceptance of public clinics for families of all income levels, but also because of the policies of health insurance programs. The latter often do not cover immunizations, so that the insured family must pay personally if the infant is immunized by a personal doctor, whereas this service is free in a public health clinic. In Western European countries, therefore, the vast majority of childhood immunizations are given in public clinics.

Reporting and isolation of infectious disease cases also tend to be more complete in the welfare state settings. In part this is owing to the greater territorial coverage and a more disciplined posture of public health agencies; it is also probably due to fee claims for patient care under the insurance programs. These claims must generally indicate a diagnosis, so that an infectious case for which a fee is claimed is readily communicated to the public health authorities. In some Canadian provinces, the identification of a rheumatic fever patient through the insurance program gives a signal to public health agencies. Follow-up control of that patient with free periodic penicillin is arranged to prevent rheumatic carditis or other complications. This mechanism would not operate under the British system of capitation payment to general practitioners (i.e., without fee-for-service claims), but in Britain the long tradition of good GP relationships with local public health authorities leads to a high level of communicable disease notification.

Programs of venereal disease control in Western Europe also differ from United States patterns in certain respects. Public clinics are more highly developed, and some countries, such as Germany, mandate treatment of infectious cases under law. A person with venereal disease in a transmissable stage who does not accept therapy may be imprisoned. This happens very rarely, but the existence of such laws promotes more complete disease control. Prostitution, on the other hand, is not illegal in several Western European countries; it is, rather, subjected to surveillance through periodic examination and treatment of registered prostitutes. Such policies, however, have been changing in recent years, as the rights and dignity of women have become more equitably recognized.

Tuberculosis control in the welfare state countries differs from that in the United States principally in the legal compulsion that may be invoked on reporting and isolating cases. Mass chest x-ray surveys are sometimes offered by the health insurance socieities as a benefit of membership. The temporary disability associated with tuberculosis entitles insured workers to monetary benefits to replace lost wages in all the welfare states, a form of social insurance that in the United States is found in only a few state jurisdictions.

In the developing countries, the communicable diseases are, of course, of much higher incidence and prevalence, not only owing to the inadequacies of environmental controls but also because programs of immunization and other personal preventive services are much weaker. Because of the lesser development of public health agencies generally, and particularly at the local community level, the social security programs in Latin America often furnish preventive services to their beneficiaries. Such services may include immunizations for children and case-detection surveys for adults. Since 1938, Chile has had a Preventive Medicine Law under which insured workers receive annual chest x rays to detect tuberculosis (or other thoracic disorders) and serological tests for syphilis. With the high incidence of enteric infections in the tropics, mass campaigns for immunization against typhoid fever or cholera are also carried out in both transitional and underdeveloped countries when an epidemic of these serious communicable diseases is threatened.

Because acute communicable diseases are relatively frequent and home conditions are poor in the developing countries, special hospitals for acute infectious diseases to treat and isolate cases are commonly found. Such "pest-houses," of course, existed throughout Western Europe and the United States in earlier centuries. Isolation of a patient with an acutely contagious disease is so difficult in the typical rural village that a few isolation beds are usually also maintained in every general hospital and even in health centers.

Tuberculosis is so great a problem in nearly all the developing countries that an immunological approach, seldom applied in the industrialized countries, is often used. This is the immunization of newborn babies with BCG (bacille Calmette-Guerin) vaccine. Although there is a small risk associated with use of this product, it is much less than the later risk of contracting tuberculosis in populations where the disease is endemic. BCG vaccine is usually administered to the newborn before it leaves the institution. Because of the over-all poverty of developing countries, sanitarium facilities are seldom adequate to care for all the active tuberculosis cases, and most of them are simply kept in bed at home. Since streptomycin and other chemotherapeutic drugs have been discovered, home therapy of TB patients has become far more effective.

Venereal disease is also very prevalent in the developing countries, more so in the large cities. Prostitution is common and seldom illegal; or if it is illegal, the laws are only meagerly enforced. VD clinics are a common service at health centers, or these patients are treated along with any others coming to a health center or hospital outpatient department. Self-medication is also common, since penicillin can be quite freely purchased at pharmacies, either for oral use or injection by the pharmacist. Cultural or religious attitudes seldom permit sex education in the schools of the developing countries.

Through vaccination and general improvement in sanitation, smallpox has been so reduced throughout the world that it has been essentially eradicated everywhere except in a few extremely underdeveloped countries. Mass campaigns to vaccinate almost total national populations have, therefore, been mounted over the last decade in certain African and Asian countries with the assistance of the World Health Organization. In 1975 a case of smallpox, found in Bangladesh and treated, was declared by WHO to be the last case on earth of this once rampant disease.

As discussed earlier, malaria, schistosomiasis, and other vector-borne communicable diseases have been tackled in the developing countries mainly through environmental measures. Leprosy is another disease, largely confined to the very poor developing countries, the control of which has depended on institutionalization and treatment of cases. Contrary to popular belief, leprosy is not highly contagious but is spread through prolonged interpersonal contacts under very insanitary conditions. The general approach to control has been isolation of patients in special leper colonies, and in many developing countries such places accommodate more cases than do tuberculosis sanitariums. Popular dread of the person who has once been infected with leprosy is so great that, even if the disease process has been arrested with drug therapy, these patients generally remain isolated for life.

In the socialist countries, the control or prevention of communicable diseases is generally part of the over-all health service program of health centers. Immunizations are given to infants soon after childbirth. When new vaccines have been discovered, such as those against poliomyelitis or measles, campaigns are launched rapidly to immunize every child in the land at health centers or schools. In Cuba, for example, a few years after its 1959 Revolution, a mass campaign to immunize the total population was launched; poliomyelitis declined precipitously from 342 reported cases in 1961 to none in 1965. One case occurring in 1970 was evidently brought in by an immigrant. Likewise, a diphtheria immunization campaign, starting in 1963, resulted in a decline from 923 cases in that year to seven in 1970.

Housing conditions in the Soviet Union and other socialist countries are still much more crowded than in the welfare states (except perhaps Japan) and the United States. Yet tuberculosis, so intimately associated with poor housing, has been greatly reduced by case detection, isolation, and treatment of cases. In Cuba, the TB death rate was reduced from 19.6 per 100,000 in 1962 to 7.3 in 1970—a decline proportionately much greater than in other Latin American countries during so short a time.

The campaigns against venereal disease in the socialist countries illustrate well the relationship of preventive services to general social and political ideology. Prostitution has been regarded as an evil of capitalism, causing both degradation of women and the spread of venereal infection. In both Russia and China, soon after their socialist revolutions, brothels were closed down and prostitutes were placed in programs of rehabilitation. In addition to medical treatment, they received training for productive employment and general education. Anyone who reopened a brothel or served as a procurer was severely punished. All VD cases were treated in health centers or polyclinics, and epidemiological follow-up of contacts was vigorously pursued. As a result of these policies, it is claimed that syphilis has been virtually wiped out, and gonorrhea has been reduced to very low rates in these countries.

In the People's Republic of China, a mass campaign that involves both environmental efforts and personal disease control has been the fight against "the four pests"—mosquitoes, flies, bedbugs, and rats. In addition to larvicidal efforts in mosquito-breeding swamps and spraying dwellings with DDT, children are given small awards for killing these vermin by hand. A bottle full of dead flies, for example, entitles the child to a prize. By such simple methods of vector control, many infectious diseases have been greatly reduced in China.

Maternal and Child Health Services

All countries emphasize preventive services for expectant mothers and small children. It is not simply that these groups have strong emotional appeal but also that the potentialities of prevention are great in the prenatal and early childhood periods. Moreover, health protection in the early years has an influence on health status throughout life. Promotion of sound nutrition, prevention of childhood infections that might cause permanent blindness or deafness, protection against numerous communicable diseases, even child-rearing practices, have a great bearing on adult physical and mental health. In no health service sector is the aphorism about an ounce of prevention being worth a pound of cure more valid than in the preventive services extended to mothers and children.

The features of these maternal and child health (MCH) services, nevertheless, differ greatly among the several types of health care system. In the free enterprise setting, they are primarily a matter of private care from individual doctors. Numerous public MCH clinics have been established, especially for preventive service to infants, but they are used by only a small fraction of the population. The proportion of newborn babies seen in health department clinics of the United States during a year is estimated to vary from 10 to 20 percent. The rest are seen by private doctors or not preventively attended at all.

The private medical profession in the United States has been so politically strong that health departments, which offer organized MCH services, lean over backward to avoid being competitive with private doctors. They do this basically by confining their services to prevention, and they underscore this intent by defining their programs as well-baby clinics; some even shun the term *clinic* by speaking of well-child conferences. If the baby is sick, a private doctor is to be consulted or, if the patient is too poor, a hospital outpatient department.

Only after 1965, when American doctors had become extremely busy and affluent and when the problems of access to medical care by the poor had become critical, was there any significant change in this exclusively preventive approach. Federal funds were provided for establishing comprehensive maternity and infant care (MIC) clinics, in selected poor neighborhoods, where treatment could be given to the sick child, as well as preventive measures to the well child. Similar comprehensive clinics were also organized for children and youth

(CY) in poor districts. These integrated preventive and therapeutic units under government auspices, however, are exceptional, and the vast majority of MCH services in the United States are purely preventive in orientation.

The same cautious approach applies to health services offered in the schools of the United States. A school nurse may be on the premises for health education purposes and first aid in case of injuries. The children may be periodically examined by a school doctor, or their vision and hearing may be tested by the nurse or audiologist. If any disorders are detected, however, the parents are typically sent a message to take the child to a personal doctor. Only if later follow-up reveals that the child's condition has not been treated is it customary for the school or public health authorities to intervene and arrange needed care, such as provision of eyeglasses.

In a few matters, the free enterprise United States has intercepted personal freedom by legally mandating certain MCH procedures. Most states, for example, require premarital serological testing to detect syphilis to prevent the birth of congenitally syphilitic babies. It has also long been required by state laws that newborn babies get antiseptic drops (silver nitrate, usually) instilled in their eyes to prevent eye infections during the birth process. Testing of newborn urine for phenylketonuria has also been mandated by many state laws to detect a rare metabolic disorder that leads to mental retardation but that can be prevented by a special diet. All these procedures, however, are typically carried out by private health personnel.

In the welfare states, organized MCH services tend to be more highly developed. In Great Britain and the Scandinavian countries, the vast majority of newborn babies are seen at official child health stations that are by no means limited to the poor but serve 80 to 90 percent of the families. Services are still preventive, with the sick child usually being referred to the family doctor, but there is no hesitation to treat minor illness. Under the Western European health insurance programs, doctors are so busy that they do not look upon these public services as competitive. In fact, in the British setting with capitation payment to general practitioners, the public MCH clinics are so crowded that special fees are offered to GPs to encourage their giving immunizations and thereby lightening the load on the public clinics. In France, attendance at the public child health clinics is encouraged by the social security program; children's allowances (small monthly grants to the mother for each child) are a regular benefit of French Social Security (as in about sixty-five countries), but they are started only when the mother brings proof that her baby has been taken to a child health clinic.

Much of the service in child health clinics is given by nurses who are specially trained for this work; in addition to learning about infant feeding and other preventive counseling, these nurses learn to detect abnormalities that warrant referral of the child to a doctor. Sometimes the clinics are scheduled with a nurse in attendance daily, while a doctor comes perhaps one or two sessions a week. Tradition, of course, plays its part, as illustrated in New Zealand, where the MCH program is conducted largely by the voluntary Royal New Zealand Society for the Health of Women and Children, better known as the Plunket Society. Since 1907, this society has been conducting preventive clinics for both prenatal and infant health guidance through a combination of volunteer services and government subsidy to pay full-time nurses. In 1965, over 92 percent of newborn babies were supervised at Plunket facilities. In Japan, preventive MCH services are given at a network of government health centers constructed after World War II.

Health examinations of school children are quite systematically carried out in the Western European welfare states. Although payment for these services is often made by the educational authorities, the work is usually done by personnel of the health department. Since dental disease is a major problem in this age group, many welfare state countries put special emphasis on school dental programs that are both preventive and curative. The strategy of the New Zealand dental nurse has been discussed earlier in connection with health manpower. In the Scandinavian countries, fully trained dentists on salary work in the schools and serve all the children. Since these countries have produced an exceptionally high ratio of dentists, it has not been difficult to recruit them for this type of work—a problem encountered in Great Britain, France, and other countries.

Maternal and child health services are also emphasized in the public health programs of the developing countries of both types. Infant mortality rates (deaths in the first year of life per 1,000 live births) have typically been so high in these countries that the benefits of preventive MCH efforts are particularly prominent. Therefore, the major activity of most health centers operated by ministries of health in Asia, Africa, or Latin America is usually health service to expectant mothers and small children.

With the meager supplies of doctors in the developing countries, nearly all MCH services are provided by nursing personnel who are often assistant nurses rather than fully trained registered nurses. The babies are immunized by these nurses, and the mothers are given advice on breast feeding and preparation of nutritious infant foods. If the child is sick, there is no hesitation to give treatment at a health center, although the decision on any drugs to be prescribed is made by a male medical assistant or sometimes a doctor. In the larger cities, MCH clinics will often have a doctor on hand, but only infrequently is there a doctor in the small towns or villages. On the other hand, where a city hospital is nearby, the seriously sick child will often be referred to the hospital outpatient department.

Gastroenteritis is extremely common in infants in the developing countries and is a major cause of death. The dehydration and malnutrition that result from prolonged diarrhea can be fatal. To cope with this, a rehydration service, giving parenteral glucose and saline infusions to infants for several days, is offered in health centers without regular hospitalization. Childhood disease is also caused by protein deprivation, especially after the small child is weaned. A major task, therefore, is to provide the nutritional education and economic support for children's diets which will include protein, even if it is derived from vegetable sources.

School health services are quite deficient in the developing countries. Outside the main cities, examinations of school children are seldom done. If nurses from the public health agency visit the schools, it is usually to give immunizations and some health education on hygienic habits.

Only in the socialist countries are the preventive and treatment services to mothers and children fully integrated. Since health centers and polyclinics, staffed by full-time salaried doctors and nurses, are the regular mode for delivery of ambulatory treatment services, these facilities provide the preventive services as well. For administrative as well as technical reasons, clinic sessions for normal babies or expectant mothers may be scheduled at certain times each week, but these sessions are staffed by the same doctors and nurses who treat the child or mother at times of sickness. (The principal reason for holding separate preventive sessions is to avoid spreading infections from a sick child and to permit convenient handling of routine procedures such as weighing and measuring babies by nurses. There is no issue of avoiding competition with private doctors.)

In the Soviet Union and some countries influenced by it, medical education puts special stress on the training of pediatricians. Pediatrics is regarded not as a specialty but as general practice for children, and training for it begins after the second year of the six-year medical curriculum. Thus, there is a particularly large number of pediatricians in the Soviet Union, enough to conduct routine examinations of all children both in the health centers and the schools.

Infant mortality rates have long been regarded as a sensitive indicator of the standard of living of a country. The rates are influenced, of course, by general environmental conditions, levels of nutrition, standards of housing, the education level of mothers, as well as the availability of specific health services, both preventive and curative. It has been a source of much concern in recent years, therefore, that the infant mortality rate of the United States has been higher than that of some fifteen to twenty other nations. Since these are all industrially advanced countries, with effective public health systems, the difference cannot be attributed to failures in reporting or other statistical artifacts. Moreover, the *average* standard of living in the United States is believed to be the highest in the world, even though there are marked variations within the country. The differentials, therefore, would seem to be due, at least in part, to inadequacies in the child health services, both preventive and therapeutic. Although these inadequacies may be concentrated in certain low-income social classes, the point is that poor populations in other countries are evidently better served by MCH services and other components of the health care system.

Family Planning Programs

Closely related to maternal and child health services are the mounting activities in many countries to promote contraception and to control the size of families. The topic of family planning and population policy is beyond the scope of this book, and here we may simply note some organizational aspects of these efforts.

Methods other than sexual abstinence of preventing conception after intercourse have been known and advocated for at least a century. Malthus published his famous essay about the dangers of population growth in 1798. In 1877, the use of contrceptives was publicly advocated in England; the legal prosecution of its promoters led to the formation of a Malthusian League. It was the work, however, of an American visiting nurse in New York City, Margaret Sanger, that launched the birth control movement in 1914 and initiated the now worldwide organized efforts to disseminate knowledge and promote the use of contraception.

Contraceptive devices of many sorts have been widely known since the early twentieth century. They have generally been available from private doctors to the more educated and affluent families of almost every country. About 1920 it became widely recognized that low-income people, in greatest need of this knowledge to avoid the hardships of excessively large families, were least able to get it. Hence, there were started in the United States and Europe special clinics to give advice, instruction, and materials for contraception or, what is now more generally called, family planning.

Because of religious objections to artificial interference with the "natural law" and associated legal obstacles, open public clinics for the purpose of family planning have been very controversial in many countries. The World Health Organization did not consider the matter sufficiently acceptable politically to launch a program in this field until 1965—and then only with the label of human reproduction studies. In nations under strong Catholic influence, family planning service must still be obtained in clandestine ways, although this is seldom a problem for affluent families.

Most countries, however, now conduct organized programs of family planning service and recognize their importance both for promoting individual family welfare and for national population control. Although the earth's potential for producing food (with the capabilities of crop rotation, fertilizer, irrigation, agricultural machinery, etc.) is far greater than Malthus predicted, it has become increasingly recognized that there must be some limits and, moreover, that large populations face problems other than a scarcity of food. The differences among countries concern chiefly the manner in which family planning activities are organized.

Family planning (FP) services in the United States follow a wide variety of patterns. Although FP started in special clinics set up exclusively for this purpose, it has increasingly been incorporated as part of the regular MCH programs of health departments. The majority of American women, however, see private doctors and get FP instruction and advice from them. For men, condoms are available over the counter at any pharmacy. Hospitals with maternity departments often furnish FP services on the woman's request after a childbirth. Thousands of special clinics also still operate, and FP services are usually regarded as a routine part of the program of gynecology clinics in hospital outpatient departments, of student health programs at universities, and of other health care arrangements. When provided under health department auspices, FP services are usually free, but most other modes require some payment for the service.

In the welfare states, there are great variations in FP information depending on religious influences. Italy, for example, did not until very recently sanction public clinics, whereas the Protestant Scandinavian countries offer FP services widely through their public health programs. In most countries with national health insurance, however, FP service is conventionally available from general medical practitioners as a normal insurance benefit. Because of this and because general practitioners are proportionately in larger supply than in the United States, public clinics are not so necessary in Western Europe, although they exist for promotional purposes.

The most prominent thrust of FP activities since about 1950 has been in the developing countries where population growth has been accelerated owing to a marked reduction in death rates. As a result, the demands for food and other resources have exceeded the capacities of these economies to produce them. The greatest prominence has been given to FP efforts in India where the population problem, combined with an economy of very low productivity, has been especially serious. With much international assistance, virtually the entire structure of official health services in India has been recast to incorporate FP services at every stage. Even the name of the central public health authority was changed to the Ministry of Health and Family Planning. The technical aspects and demographic outcomes of these efforts are discussed elsewhere in this volume, but here we may simply note that the administrative approach has been through integration of FP activities into the over-all system of health services.

In nearby Malaysia, on the other hand, FP activities have been promoted by a special unit in the office of the prime minister, rather than through the Malaysian Ministry of Health. Personnel under a separate budget do this work, rather than the regular complement of public health nurses and others. The health centers and hospitals of the Ministry of Health provide space for FP clinics, but they are conducted by the special FP workers at hours different from those of regular MCH or other public health clinics. This separate administrative pattern has been applied in many countries for religious or political reasons. Sometimes the sponsorship is ostensibly by a nonofficial association, which receives most of its funds from the government.

In Africa, the problem of overpopulation has not been perceived so seriously as in Asia. FP activities, however, have been increasingly incorporated in the scope of services offered by the regular governmental MCH programs. Latin American countries, with their Catholic heritage, have been slow to develop FP programs until very recently. Objections by the church, however, have been receding, and in Chile, Panama, and a few other countries FP services are being sponsored by voluntary societies and offered at ministry of health facilities. The low availability of contraceptive techniques, however, has led to a very high rate of illegal abortion in many Latin American countries.

The socialist countries have shown changing attitudes to birth control and abortion, in step with their population policies. Soon after its 1917 revolution, the Soviet Union made contraceptive information and devices freely available as a routine aspect of the health service. Abortion was also legalized to prevent criminal interventions, which were common and often harmful or fatal throughout Europe. Then in 1936, after FP services had become widely disseminated, excessive abortions were concluded to be harmful, and they were again prohibited except when necessary to protect the life or health of the woman. Unfortunately, clandestine abortions then rose once more (when contraception had failed), and in the 1950s the USSR legalized abortion once again. The preferred method of family planning, of course, remains contraception, which is widely promoted in the health services of all the socialist countries.

The People's Republic of China, despite its huge population, initially did not disseminate birth control information. The political leadership claimed that population control was advocated only because of the failures of capitalism to meet the needs of the people. Then, as China's population continued to grow, the limits of resources even under the socialist economy were recognized. In the 1960s, the policy was changed, and FP services were widely promoted both as an instrument of population control and as a measure for the liberation of women. Today FP instruction and devices are given by every barefoot doctor and at all health centers. Socialist propaganda favors late marriage in China and families with no more than two or three children.

Other Preventive Programs

Health education of the population is an aspect of many preventive programs, but in some countries the promotion of such activities has become a special professional discipline. Perhaps it is because the general field of mass communication is so highly developed in the United States as an aspect of commercial advertising that health education developed first here as a formal function of health departments.

A major thrust of health education in the United States came with the venereal disease campaign of the 1930s. It was important that these diseases, long hidden in secrecy, should be brought out into the open, so that cases could be detected and treated. Posters, films, talks, pamphlets, radio programs—all sorts of mass media were used to spread the message. It soon became clear that more than communication was required, and health education evolved into a technique for the organization of people to work on community health problems—whether VD or tuberculosis, accidents, malnutrition, the need for prenatal care, or anything else. As other health problems have become more prominent, health educational efforts have been beamed at heart disease, cancer detection, alcoholism, cigarette smoking and lung cancer, drug abuse, family planning, and almost every medical topic.

Largely through American influence, this approach to health promotion or disease prevention has been spread throughout the world. In a sense, the approach is built on a libertarian philosophy, through which persuasion is emphasized in contrast to law or compulsion. To some extent, this philosophy has been adopted by every type of country, but some contrasts may be noted. The British, for example, attempt to educate people about the harmfulness of excessive alcohol and tobacco; but at the same time they have imposed very high excise taxes on these products—much higher than those in America—and the reduction in alcoholism and tobacco consumption has been dramatic. Health education in Western Europe, moreover, is considered an aspect of the work of all public health personnel and is seldom a special professional discipline.

Similarly, in the developing countries, health education techniques are used as tools in campaigns to control malaria, reduce infant mortality, improve nutritional practices, and promote family planning. At the national level, posters and pamphlets may be printed and films produced, but only rarely is a trained health educator on the staff of a local public health unit. In rural areas of developing countries, health films are an especially popular strategy, since so little other local entertainment is ordinarily available, but they are shown by sanitarians or nurses. Widespread illiteracy is an obstacle to using much in the way of health literature. The schools, however, often include hygiene instruction in their curricula.

In the Soviet Union and China, health education is regarded as a task of every doctor and nurse. At hospitals and health centers, one sees posters or movies on many health topics. The health lesson is often combined with a political message. When typhus fever was endemic in postrevolutionary Russia, Lenin was frequently quoted: "Socialism must defeat the louse, or the louse will defeat socialism." Modern China's attacks on the "four pests," already noted, are defined as patriotic health campaigns.

Preventive health services at workplaces have mounted as industrialization has increased. The field of occupational medicine is best developed, therefore, in the most highly industrialized countries, where the risks of work accidents and occupational diseases are great. In the welfare states, where labor unions are strong and protective social legislation has long been in effect, government supervision of working conditions is strict. As part of the ministry of labor, there is typically a factory inspection service (including a medical inspector of factories or mines) with more rigorous standards than characterize similar practices in the United States. It was only in 1972, that the United States enacted the first federal Occupational Safety and Health Act (OSHA); before then, surveillance of safety and toxic substances at workplaces was left up to each of the states, and in many it was extremely lax. Even the federal OSHA program has only a fraction of the staffing necessary to do the job and remains proportionately much weaker than both the inspection and enforcement programs in most European countries.

In every country, the greatest difficulties in preventing occupational accidents and diseases occur in small plants. Worker's compensation legislation, with its experience rating (according to the accident frequency) of insurance premiums paid by employers, has been generally effective in inducing large enterprises to have safety measures (guarded machinery, protective work clothing, rest periods, etc.), as well as in-plant health services. In small plants, such precautions are seldom undertaken because of their costs unless there is government pressure. However, in the developing countries, most working establishments are relatively small and would be very difficult to control even if the ministry of labor were strong. In the economically advanced countries, too, a large fraction of workers are employed in small plants, but government controls are more diligent. Soon after World War II, France enacted unusual mandatory legislation for in-plant health services. To meet legal requirements, groups of small plants in many cities have developed cooperative industrial health service programs that none of the individual plants could afford alone.

The socialist countries accord a very high priority to the health of industrial workers. In-plant health services are not limited to protection against work hazards but often include the provision of any type of medical care needed by the worker. The rates of sickness absenteeism must be reported to government authorities, and a high rate provides the signal for investigation and perhaps corrective action. Unlike the Western European pattern, in Eastern European countries the supervision of industrial safety and health is a responsiblity of the ministries of health.

As the major causes of morbidity and death have shifted in the advanced industrial countries from the communicable diseases to the degenerative disorders of later life, efforts have increased to apply preventive techniques to these conditions. In large part, this effort has depended on epidemiological research to discover the circumstances causing or contributing to such diseases as cancer, hypertension, cardiovascular disease, arthritis, diabetes, and many other afflictions. Most of this research has been conducted in the United States, Great Britain, Germany, and a few other industrialized countries.

Even when contributory factors to the genesis of a chronic disease are discovered, the implementation of a preventive program is not so easy. The role of cigarette smoking in causing lung cancer, for example, has been well established, but the actions taken so far in the United States have had only minor effects. Cigarette packages must be labeled as being hazardous to health, television advertising of cigarettes has been banned, taxes on cigarettes have been raised, antismoking clinics have been set up, and all sorts of health education campaigns have been launched. Individual behavior, however, has been difficult to influence, as long as cigarettes provide certain pleasures and are manufactured in the billions. Similar difficulties confront the effort to educate people about obesity and diabetes and the consumption of saturated fats and arteriosclerosis. The difficulties are compounded by uncertainties about the epidemiological truths.

In the absence of clear-cut knowledge about primary prevention of the noncommunicable diseases, public health authorities in the United States have promoted screening procedures, that is, secondary prevention by which a disease may be detected at an early incipient stage before it is causing overt symptoms. When a battery of several such tests is given, it is called multiphasic screening, and this may be done in various public settings. Cytological tests for early signs of uterine cancer ("Pap smears") or blood glucose tests for early signs of diabetes are common screening procedures widely undertaken in the United States. Public health scientists in Western Europe, however, especially in Great Britain, are not so sure about the value of this strategy; they question whether early detection of a disorder and its early treatment will affect the ultimate outcome. To launch these tests on a nationwide scale would, of course, be expensive in manpower and equipment. For the present, therefore, multiphasic screening has not been adopted as a general preventive strategy in any of the welfare states.

In the developing countries, screening tests for the noncommunicable diseases have not been widely used because of their costs and because other measures of prevention have higher priority. The well-to-do can sometimes get a battery of tests performed in a private hospital, but such tests are not provided as general public health policy.

The Soviet Union encourages periodic health examinations of the whole population, with special emphasis on the young, on women in the child-bearing years, and on workers in high-risk occupations. This policy, called dispensarization, involves a few laboratory tests of urine and blood, but is principally a clinical examination. Education about the hazards of cigarette smoking does not even constitute a part of the preventive health programs of the USSR or the People's Republic of China. On a world scale, it would seem that there is no general consensus on ways to prevent the chronic and noninfectious diseases through organized measures.

Readings

Banerji, D., *Family Planning in India: A Critique and A Perspective*, New Delhi: People's Publishing House, 1971.

Behrman, S. J., Leslie Corsa, Jr., and Roland Freeman (eds.), *Fertility and Family Planning: A World View*, Ann Arbor: University of Michigan Press, 1969.

Board, L. M., "Problems and Priorities in Combatting Air, Water, and Soil Pollution in Developing Countries," *Archives of Environmental Health, 18*:260-264 (February 1969).

Brockington, Fraser, *World Health*, London: Penguin Books, 1958.

David, Henry P. (ed.), *International Trends in Mental Health*, New York: McGraw-Hill Book Co., 1966.

Furman, Sylvan S., *Community Mental Health Services in Northern Europe: Great Britain, Netherlands, Denmark, and Sweden*, Washington, D.C.: U.S. National Institute of Mental Health, 1965.

Gittelman, Martin, "Coordinating Mental Health Systems: A National and International Perspective," *American Journal of Public Health, 64*:496-500 (May 1974).

Gonzalez, C. L., *Mass Campaigns and General Health Services*, Geneva: World Health Organization, Public Health Papers No. 29, 1965.

Holmes, A. C., *Health Education in Developing Countries*, London: Thomas Nelson and Sons, 1964.

Horn, Joshua, *Away with All Pests: An English Surgeon in People's China 1954-1969*, New York: Monthly Review Press, 1971.

Kessler, Alexander and C. C. Standley, "Health, Family Planning, and Population Growth," *International Journal of Health Services, 3*:561-566 (1973).

King, Maurice et al., *Nutrition for Developing Countries*, Nairobi: Oxford University Press, 1973.

Kohner, A., "The Impact of Public Health Programs on Economic Development," *International Journal of Health Services, 1*:285-292 (August 1971).

Lambo, T. A., "Planning and Organization of Public Health Facilities in Africa," *Journal of Social Health of Nigeria, 6*:186-194 (1971).

Lapham, Robert J. and W. Parker Maudlin, "National Family Planning Programs: Review and Evaluation," *Studies in Family Planning, 3*:29-52 (March 1972).

Parker, Julia, *Local Health and Welfare Services*, London: George Allen and Unwin, 1965.

Paul, Benjamin D., *Health, Culture, and Community*, New York: Russel Sage Foundation, 1955.

Polgar, Steven and Alexander Kessler, *An Introduction to Family Planning in the Context of Health Services*, Geneva: World Health Organization, 1968.

Raulet, H. M., "Family Planning and Population Control in Developing Countries," *Demography, 7*:211-234 (May 1970).

Roemer, Milton I., "Health Departments and Medical Care: A World Scanning," *American Journal of Public Health, 50*:154-160 (February 1960).

Rosen, George, *A History of Public Health,* New York: MD Publications, 1958.

Rosselot, J., "Maternal and Child Health in Latin America," *Boletin de la Oficina Sanitaria Panamericana* (English Edition), *6*:21-32 (1972).

Thorner, Robert M. et al., "A Study to Evaluate the Effectiveness of Multiphasic Screening in Yugoslavia," *Preventive Medicine, 2*:295-301 (1973).

Wagner, E. G. and J. N. Lanoix, *Excreta Disposal for Rural Areas and Small Communities,* Geneva: World Health ORganization, 1958.

Walsh, J., "International Patterns of Oral Health Care—The Example of New Zealand," *New Zealand Dental Journal, 66*:143-152 (April 1970).

Williams, Cicely D. and Derrick B. Jelliffe, *Mother and Child Health: Delivering the Services,* London: Oxford University Press, 1972.

World Health Organization, Regional Office for Europe, *Public Health Administration in Europe,* Copenhagen: WHO, 1965.

World Health Organization, Expert Committee on Dental Health, *Organization of Dental Public Health Services,* Geneva: WHO, Tech. Report Series No. 298, 1965.

World Health Organization, *Nutrition: A Review of the W.H.O. Programme 1965-1971,* Geneva: WHO, 1972.

Zarour, George I., "Considerations on Basic Aspects of School Health Education in Developing Countries," *International Journal of Health Education, 14*: 90-99 (1971).

8

HEALTH CARE REGULATION

As health care systems have become more complex, involving more people and greater expenditures of funds, regulation through various social processes has become increasingly necessary to assure that investments of effort and resources are kept "on track" toward their intended objectives.

A definition of *regulation* is not easy, since almost any social action may exert an influence, direct or indirect, on the behavior of people. This chapter will, however, employ the concept in a relatively modest or restricted sense. First, we will examine the regulatory influences, both governmental and voluntary, on the preparation of health manpower and their legal authorization to serve the population in various types of country. Next, we will consider the regulation of other types of health care resource, particularly health facilities and drugs. Third, we will review briefly the different ways that the continuing performance of personnel is monitored under various health care systems.

Regulation of Health Personnel

To assure or attempt to achieve a certain quality of services in a health care system, there are numerous methods of regulation of the qualifications of health personnel. The policies vary among the types of country and for different categories of health profession or occupation.

Free Enterprise Systems

In the free enterprise setting, government licensure of physicians and many (though not all) other forms of personnel is the basic approach to regulation of health manpower. Licensure of the health professions is highly diversified among the American federation of fifty state jurisdictions. In California, as many as twenty one different health service disciplines are subject to licensure under the State Department of Consumer Affairs. There are eleven health fields that are licensed in some form in all fifty states, although the type of state agency varies. The smallest number of different health occupations subject to licensure is in Iowa and four other states, where twelve fields are licensed.

The American policy on licensure of physicians reflects the consequences of a free enterprise ideology with respect to educational institutions. Since universities and medical schools were (until the 1910-1920 period) essentially free from governmental or any other regulation, the state authorities could not depend on the quality of training. As a result, special state medical examinations were required for licensure, a practice that is relatively uncommon around the world. The first such state law was enacted in Texas in 1873, followed soon by all the other states. In most states, the members of the medical examining board are chosen by the governor from nominations submitted by the private state medical association; only in recent years have nonphysician members been appointed to these boards as a hedge against the promotion of the commercial self-interest of doctors.

Reciprocity gradually grew among the states in recognition of one anothers' licensees; today this permits mobility of doctors among about 75 percent of the states. In 1915 a nongovernmental National Board of Medical Examiners was formed; this voluntary body offers a relatively rigorous three-part examination (basic sciences, clinical fields, and practical aspects) that is accepted by all but a few states. In 1966 about three-fourths of the nation's medical schools required their students to take the first two parts of this examination. The fifty state examining boards have also cooperated recently in establishing a uniform examination prepared by the Federation of Licensure Examining Boards (FLEX) to achieve technical uniformity. The FLEX examination has been especially useful in licensure of foreign medical graduates, whose numbers have greatly increased since the immigration law changes of 1948. In addition to the examination, state boards may require internships and other credentials. There is also a nongovernmental Educational Commission for Foreign Medical Graduates (ECFMG) which offers a test both overseas and in the United States as a screening procedure for foreign graduates who intend to seek postgraduate training or restricted employment (e.g., in a mental hospital) in an American state.

The specialties in medicine have been subject only to nongovernmental regulation in the free enterprise United States setting. Under the pressure of competition from nonphysician optometrists, the first United States specialty board was established in 1915 in the field of ophthalmology. Gradually, additional specialty boards, establishing criteria for training as well as for formal examinations, were founded and became affiliated eventually with the American Medical Association. Today there are about twenty principal boards for certifying specialty competence and an additional fifteen subspecialty disciplines (e.g., cardiology as a subdivision of internal medicine). It is noteworthy that, although it is nationwide in operation and impact, this regulatory program is not governmental. Yet, specialty board certification is recognized for participation and payment purposes by many government programs (e.g., the state crippled children's services) and by most hospitals for staff appointments. However, there is no law requiring specialty board certification as a condition for engaging in various types of medical practice—for example, surgery or radiology. Hospitals may establish their own rules for physician appointment or definition of professional "privileges," but these are not statutory.

As mentioned in an earlier chapter, the most recent specialty in the American medical scene is family practice, designed to increase the training and status of generalists. This is also the only specialty field now requiring periodic recertification; a family practice specialist must take every five years a certain amount of continuing education to reestablish his specialty status. For maintenance of over-all medical licensure, the state of New Mexico has also mandated a minimum amount of continuing education each five years since 1970, and a number of other states are now following its example. Only in this way, it is argued, can the population be assured that a doctor is keeping informed on new advances in medical science.

Most other health science disciplines in the United States have followed the model of medicine in their state licensure requirements, but there are a number of noteworthy variations. Dentistry, for example, has a statutory rather than a purely voluntary basis for specialty status in several states. Registration of trained nurses requires a formal examination in every state, but a national federation has established one uniform set of questions. As a result, reciprocity in recognition of RN qualifications is universal among the fifty states. Examinations in pharmacy are also required in all states, and in twelve jurisdictions relicensure is periodically required on the basis of a minimum record of continuing education.

Some health professions are not required to have government licensure at all in certain states, for example, laboratory technology. In those states mandating licensure, the candidate must usually pass an examination in addition to having credentials from an approved school. In the other states, the laboratory technologist or technician may simply offer to prospective employers a voluntary credential: certification by the American Society of Clinical Pathologists, which is based on having attended a school approved by the Society and having passed its examination. Certain new health disciplines, such as inhalation therapy, are licensed in only a few states, as is true of clinical psychology. Hospital administration is a field defined as subject to state licensure in only one state, Minnesota. On the other hand, nursing home administration is the first field that, by national law, requires state licensure (meeting minimal requirements) under certain conditions. Serious deficiencies were detected in the administration of nursing homes serving patients under the federal Medicare program, and the national requirement was imposed as a corrective action. Nursing homes are reimbursed for Medicare patients only if they are headed by licensed administrators.

Although the state licensure of health professions in the United States is highly variable, several voluntary professional societies have attempted to fill some regulatory gaps. Nonofficial approval of various types of auxiliary personnel, such as pharmacy or laboratory assistants, is being offered by the corresponding national societies, based on examinations or proof of satisfactory training. Probably more important is the role of these societies in the approval or accreditation of educational programs. Since neither state nor federal governments have taken initiative in approving professional training programs, it is being done by the private societies. The roles of the American Medical Association and the Association of American Medical Colleges in approving medical schools have been noted previously. The same sort of approval has been carried out by the American Pharmaceutical Association with respect to schools of pharmacy, the National League for Nursing regarding schools of professional nursing (i.e., those offering R.N. awards), and so on. There is, furthermore, a National Commission on Accrediting, another voluntary body, which helps to establish general criteria for reviewing educational programs in all fields. Finally, in the federal U.S. Office of Education there is a unit, recently formed, to approve the accrediting associations; only at this point has government entered the picture.

Welfare State Systems

The diversity of patterns of regulating health manpower in the many welfare states is too great to permit anything but a few examples. In general (with several notable exceptions), one finds that in these countries greater control is exercised by national governments over the educational programs. As a result, the establishment of qualifications for engaging in various forms of health service is usually much simpler than in the United States. Proof of graduation from a government approved training program usually grants the legal right to engage in the profession more or less automatically.

In Sweden or Norway, for example, all the medical schools must be approved by the national Ministry of Education or its equivalent. Then a medical graduate need only present his credentials to the health authorities in the national Ministry of Social Affairs (Norway) for registration. In these countries, the same procedure applies to nurses, except that the maintenance of registration records has been delegated by the government to the voluntary nurses association. In France and West Germany, the basic government controls apply also to the educational institutions. No further examination is required of medical graduates.

In Germany, the new graduate must then have two years of hospital training, after which registration with a provincial (not national) health authority becomes a pro forma matter. In France, the new medical graduate simply registers, on the basis of his academic credentials, with the local government (prefect) in the area where he settles. For ethical and professional surveillance, he must also register with the national *Ordre des Medicins* (Order of Physicians). Similar policies are followed in Belgium and Holland.

Great Britain differs slightly from most welfare states in requiring its medical schools and their examinations to be approved by the General Medical Council, a prestigious voluntary body, even though all the educational institutions are also approved and supervised by the Ministry of Education. Canada even requires that the graduate pass a national examination given by the Medical Council of Canada. It is claimed that this second examination does not reflect distrust of the schools but rather is intended to help them maintain their standards. In Great Britain, there are still further examination hurdles that are, however, voluntary. These examinations are for fellowship in the Royal College of Physicians or the Royal College of Surgeons, and they are more rigorous and specialized examinations. Passing them entitles the doctor to add FRCP or FRCS after his name, as a mark of additional status and competence.

Japan illustrates the influence of politics on regulatory processes. Before World War II, Japan followed the German model of automatic registration of medical and other health science graduates after schooling, relying on supervision of the schools by the national educational authorities. Then during the postwar occupation by United States armed forces, the American pattern of a second examination was imposed. Some years later, great resistance to this came from the students, and the prewar policies were reinstated.

Generally speaking, the procedures for licensure or registration of nurses, pharmacists, and other health personnel follow the model of physicians in each country. There may be slight modifications in certain fields—as in Norway where, although there is no second examination of nursing graduates by the government, the final examination administered by each nursing school consists of a nationally uniform set of questions.

Verification of specialty status in medicine varies among the welfare states, although it is primarily left up to professional bodies. In France, there are two classes of specialist: (1) those who are devoted exclusively to a specialty, or *médecins specialsts* and (2) those engaging in a specialty but also continuing with some general practice, or *médecins compétents*. Both types are so registered with the Ministry of National Education after completing appropriate training and passing examinations given by the several specialty societies. They are also so registered in each *département* or province. In Norway, the national medical association simply maintains a committee that regulates specialty training requirements and gives examinations. In Belgium, there are no examinations, but an especially rigorous sequence of training is required in every field, and it must be approved in advance by the national medical association. If the medical candidate passes through all the stages successfully, he is awarded specialty credentials by the medical association. In Belgium and indeed in most welfare state countries, specialty status must be registered with a government authority if the doctor is then to be entitled to payments from the health insurance program at higher specialist rates.

Less Developed and Socialist Countries

In both the transitional and the underdeveloped countries, the role of government is generally stronger and the role of the professional bodies weaker than in the welfare states. Within the Ministry of Health in Colombia, for example, there is a Council of Professional Practice which registers all physicians and other health personnel who have had prescribed training. No examination is required, but the candidate must simply show his credentials from a school recognized by the Ministry of Education; physicians must also, however, show proof of a one-year internship in a hospital plus a second year of service in a public health post or a rural facility of some type. Many Latin American countries require the latter form of service as an approach to solving the worldwide problem of rural doctor shortages. Beyond these proforma registrations, physicians, dentists, and others engaged in individual practice must usually join a professional society (*Colegio Medico de Chile,* for example) for purposes of ethical controls over their behavior. These societies may also engage in bargaining with government agencies on rates of payment for services, or they may establish parallel non-government bodies for such purposes.

In the severely underdeveloped countries, regulation of personnel tends to follow patterns laid down earlier by colonial authorities. Professional societies tend to be weak, and virtually all responsibilities are vested in ministries of health. Registration with the ministry follows automatically from completion of prescribed courses of training. Nurses and allied health personnel are registered in substantially the same way as physicians.

The socialist countries likewise require no examinations by a government authority beyond completion of specified educational programs. The Ministry of Health of Poland, for example, simply registers all nurses, physicians, and others when their training is completed. Even the educational institutions for the health disciplines are usually controlled by the national health, rather than education, authorities, so that there is no need for interchange between the two ministries of education and health. Physicians, as noted earlier, may be required to serve for two or three years in a rural area as a condition for registration. Ethical and behavioral matters are also supervised by the Polish Health Ministry.

There are nonofficial professional societies, but their functions are essentially in the field of postgraduate or continuing education. Since the over-all health care systems in the socialist countries are in structured frameworks, the hazards of malfeasance by an isolated practitioner are generally much less. Regulation is built into the course of day-to-day work.

Regulation of Other Health Care Resources

Beyond health manpower, all countries exercise some supervision over the structure of health care facilities, the production and distribution of drugs or medical supplies, and certain other inputs of the health care system.

Facility Approval

As the importance of hospitals in total health service has increased, standards for their construction and operation have increasingly been imposed by government authorities. The application of these controls varies with the over-all political ideology of countries.

In the free enterprise United States, there were very few public standards for hospital construction until the federal law to subsidize such projects was passed in 1947; as a condition for such grants to the states, each state was required to enact a hospital licensure law. Under these laws, all hospitals are periodically inspected with respect to physical standards, laboratory facilities, kitchen sanitation, fire safety, radiological protection, and related matters. Enforcement of these laws is rather weak, however, since the staffing of the state inspection authorities (usually the state department of health) is generally meager. Moreover, most of the state laws stress standards connected with the hospital's physical features and demand little in the way of standards for the functioning of the staff. Compensating for the latter, in a sense, there was established in 1950 in the United States a nongovernment body, the Joint Commission on Accreditation of Hospitals (JCAH), representing several professional associations. Accreditation by the JCAH is entirely voluntary, but it emphasizes the performance of the medical staff, the diligence of patient care, and various functional aspects of the hospital. This approval has become a generally more prestigious badge of merit than the official licensure by a state government.

Until about 1960, any hospital in the United States could be built or enlarged as long as it met state licensure requirements. As bed-population ratios increased, along with expansion of voluntary insurance for hospitalization, it became apparent that under fee-for-service medical practice almost any new beds constructed would soon become occupied by patients. In response, New York

State enacted a law in 1961 requiring that any construction providing new hospital beds had not only to meet the licensure standards but also to satisfy the state government that there was a social need for the additional beds. Such certificate of need laws were soon passed by twenty five or thrity other states. In 1974, a national law was enacted (the National Health Planning and Resource Development Act), requiring that every state must have such legislation controlling the supply of hospital beds as well as their quality standards.

Hospital construction in the welfare states has generally been more subject to government controls, although the levels of public authority differ. Voluntary accreditation bodies play no role. In British and French systems, standards for both construction and operation of hospitals are promulgated by the ministries of health at the national level, although they are monitored by regional or provincial authorities. In Great Britain, where virtually all hospitals are now actually owned and controlled by the central government, exercise of this authority is not difficult. In France, where government sponsors about 70 percent of the beds, the implementation of standards, although theoretically universal, is not so perfect for the nongovernment 30 percent. The authority in Sweden is lodged in local units of government for 95 percent of the beds, but national government standards for both construction and operation of hospitals are typically followed on a voluntary basis.

Regarding the supply or bed-population ratios of hospitals in Western Europe, the constraints becoming necessary in the free enterprise setting have not arisen. With salaried hospital doctors or, at least, selectively small hospital medical staffs, the problem of overhospitalization, with its serious cost burdens, has evidently not been felt. As a result, any local community or, in some countries, any voluntary group has been free to build hospitals, as long as they met technical standards. The high cost of construction to meet such standards is an inherent constraint.

In Canada and Japan, on the other hand, where open staff hospitals and fee remuneration of doctors for inpatient care prevail, the situation is different. After its federal-provincial hospital insurance program was enacted in 1957, Canada soon recognized that almost any beds constructed would quickly become filled with patients for whose care the entire population had to pay under the insurance system. Therefore, the provincial governments now exercise control over all new hospital construction or enlargement, requiring that there be proven a definite need for any additional beds. In fact, some provinces, faced with spiraling hospitalization costs, have even ordered the closure of certain small hospitals to limit the bed availability. Enforcement is implemented through the insurance program. In Japan, similar action has been taken recently at the national level.

In both types of developing country, the need for hospital beds has been so great and the economic resources to build them so limited that controls over quality standards and bed supply have been very limited. Many of the national ministries of health maintain technical offices to prepare architectural plans for hospitals and health centers of various sizes, along with rosters of appropriate equipment. These offices are concerned with any facilities constructed by the ministry itself (or by a ministry of public works at the request of the health authorities), and they offer advice, if requested, to private or charitable bodies building hospitals. In Latin America and several Middle East countries, some social security agencies have similar architectural design offices, but disciplinary controls are rarely exercised if a nonofficial body establishes a private hospital that does not meet central government standards. The concept seems to be that almost any sort of hospital in countries desperately short of beds is better than none.

Hospital construction in the socialist countries, being entirely governmental, presents no special problems of surveillance. Depending on the degree of centralized authority, hospitals are simply built according to the plans of the national or local government bodies. In the highly centralized model of the Soviet Union, the national Ministry of Health plans all construction or must approve projects originating at a local level (such as a collective farm), since the operating costs eventually must be met from the national health budget. In the more localized model of China or Yugoslavia, the provincial or republic authorities make their own hospital or health center construction decisions, but they may obtain advice on technical standards, if they wish, from the central health ministries.

Drug Control

The manufacture and distribution of pharmaceutical products is probably more dependent on the over-all operations of a country's economic system than any other aspect of the health services. Thus, in an essentially capitalist economy, even when the delivery of all health care has largely come under the control of government, as in the British National Health Service, the production and sale of drugs remain mainly a responsibility of private commerce.

The free enterprise ideology in American health services is especially well illustrated in the provision and distribution of drugs. Their manufacture is by private corporations, they are widely advertised to both physicians and the general population, their sale is by private pharmacists (either small merchants or corporate chains of drugstores), and their consumption depends overwhelmingly on private, noninsured payments. The harm to patients resulting from exercise of the profit motive in this field has generated a series of federal legislative responses from 1906 to 1962 that have imposed increasing controls on pharmaceutical production and distribution.

Because of the actual or potential harm done by toxic substances sold as remedies or publicized by false claims in labeling or advertising, or because of the sale of substances of unproven safety or efficacy, the Congress and many state legislatures have enacted increasingly restrictive legislation. As a result, today the United States paradoxically has more rigorous controls over drug marketing than many other countries in which the general health care system is more disciplined. In reaction to a succession of tragedies, in which patients have been poisoned or killed by innocently purchased drugs, American law now requires the manufacturer to offer rigorous proof, presented to a federal government agency, of a new product's safety as well as efficacy before it may be distributed. There is also careful surveillance of advertising claims.

Nevertheless, the freedom of hundreds of manufacturers to produce and sell their products, usually under patented brand names, results in a bewildering array of tens of thousands of drugs. Excellent university hospitals have found that a formulary or list of a few hundred preparations is adequate to deal with almost all human ailments. Yet, the free market for both production and distribution results in the sale of numerous compounds with identical chemical composition, under different names, and with widely varying prices. Moreover, there may be scores of medications with very similar pharmacological action even though their chemical composition may differ slightly or substantially. To cope with the confusion caused by this plethora of drug products, many organized health care programs have issued defined lists of drugs, often under the generic chemical name rather than the brand name, which will be financed. The generic drugs are typically less expensive. Other products may be used only at the patient's personal expense.

The social insurance programs, which usually cover prescribed drugs in the welfare states, have led to many more controls over the distribution of pharmaceutical products. In countries where few drugs are domestically manufactured, such as Norway, the legal controls over production may be relatively limited. Even in West Germany, where many drugs are manufactured, the tests mandated for drug safety have not been very strict, so that it was possible for a company to market "Thalidomide" for years, before its tragic deformative effects on the babies of pregnant women taking the drug were detected.

The marketing of drugs in the Western European countries, on the other hand, is subject to many constraints. Ministries of health, usually with the advice of expert committees of medical practitioners and pharmacologists, often issue a list of compounds that may be legally imported or sold. Such lists are periodically updated. Thus, Norway authorizes the sale of only 2,000 drugs within its borders—far fewer than the number in the United States or, in fact, West Germany. In Great Britain, the number of marketable drugs is greater, but there is a recommended list of products covered under the National Health Service; drugs not on this list and prescribed by the doctor must be paid for by the patient personally, unless the doctor can specifically justify their use in a particular case.

The Belgian social insurance program requires some cost sharing by the patient for all prescriptions, but it is a lower percentage of the price if the drug is on the officially approved list.

Pharmacies come under greater control in several welfare state systems than in the United States. In Norway, pharmacies are inspected periodically by the central government to assure their compliance with defined standards. There are also controls over the establishment of new pharmacies. In certain areas, especially the large cities, where pharmacies are abundant, new ones will not be permitted; hence, a pharmacist may be employed only in an existing pharmacy at such locations or else he must go to an underserved area if he wishes to open a new pharmacy. In Belgium, there is an unusual law placing responsibility on the dispensing pharmacist for ill effects from any prescription, even though the doctor's written orders have been accurately followed. As a result, to protect both their members and the general population, the Belgian Association of Pharmacists has long operated its own elaborate drug-testing program, over and above the controls imposed on manufacturers within Belgium by the Ministry of Health.

In the developing countries, drug controls are relatively weak. The vast majority of modern drugs are imported. Even if the packaging or the preparation of capsules, for example, is done in the country, the required chemical compounds come from outside sources. Once a company has been authorized to open a pharmaceutical plant, there is little if any government surveillance over its operation. Likewise, most drugs are readily dispensed by a pharmacy or even a general food shop with or without a prescription. There may be limitations on the sale of certain narcotics, but even these are seldom enforced. With respect to the remedies sold or administered by traditional healers in the developing countries, there are virtually no attempts at government controls. In organized programs, such as the health centers of a ministry of health or the polyclinics of a social security program, the drugs dispensed usually come from central depots and are therefore more carefully controlled.

The socialist countries control both drug production and distribution along lines parallel with the rest of their health care systems. In the Soviet Union, the number of drugs available is much smaller than in Western Europe, since only one or two compounds are produced for each pharmacological purpose. Controls are simply built into the planning of pharmaceutical production by the Ministry of Health. In the People's Republic of China, the manufacture of "western" drugs, such as antibiotics or contraceptive steroids, is planned and carried out by the Ministry of Health. The herbal drugs of traditional Chinese medicine, however, are freely produced in every local area.

Regulation of Health Care Performance

After the licensure of personnel, the approval of health facilities, or the control
of drug production and distribution, there are many further forms of regulation
feasible to assure effective performance within a health care system. These are
sometimes built into the delivery patterns, such as the discipline implicit in the
closed staff salaried doctor model of hospital organization in Europe, compared
with the open staff model with numerous private visiting doctors in the United
States. The same applies to the health center model, compared to private office
practice, for delivering ambulatory medical care. Here, however, we may examine other less direct regulatory influences: those exercised by payment
agencies, professional societies, or judicial systems.

In the United States, the laissez faire economic approach to most medical
care has led to a long-term escalation of prices; the rate of inflation has been
especially rapid over the past thirty years. Largely in response to this—although
concerns about the quality of health care also play a part—various payment
agencies have applied increasing controls. Thus, with fee-for-service payments
being used in most government programs of medical care for the poor (such as
Medicaid), many states require prior authorization by a government medical
consultant before elective surgical procedures are paid for. Such regulations, of
course, influence both the costs and the quality of the service. Other government programs, such as those for rehabilitation of disabled workers, may stipu-
late that only board-certified specialists may participate and be paid. Voluntary
health insurance programs may also review payment claims with a special eye
for abuses, such as excessive numbers of injections, diagnostic tests, or surgical
procedures of dubious value, such as tonsillectomies. On the other hand, many
voluntary insurance organizations have been criticized for being relatively loose
in their surveillance, including their exercise of the fiscal intermediary role under
the government's Medicare program for services to the aged.

Within the Medicare program, in which costs have risen very rapidly, the
federal government has been impelled to introduce more and more regulatory
constraints. The rules for determining "usual and customary" fees have become
increasingly restrictive, and legal actions have been taken against doctors sus-
pected of submitting fraudulent fee claims. In 1973, amendments to the federal
law required establishment of Professional Standard Review Organizations
(PSROs) to exercise peer review over all Medicare and Medicaid payment claims
for services in hospitals. The United States is to be covered by some 200 PSROs,
whose surveillance should, it is hoped, lead to greater self-discipline in the American medical profession.

Professional societies of physicians, dentists, nurses, and others are theoretically expected to promote ethical behavior among their members. In the
United States, nevertheless, it has been very rare for such societies to discipline

any of their members, except for the most egregious behavior, such as that associated with drug addiction, alcoholism, or frankly illegal actions. Professional societies, however, have been effective in preventing advertising by their members or other blatantly commercialized practices. On the other hand, they have often put greater energies behind political opposition to various legislative proposals that might extend health service to the population but that allegedly constrain the "freedom" of the private practitioner.

A third indirect channel of regulation is the right of the patient to take legal action against his doctor or other health care provider for injuries suffered due to negligence. In the United States, such law suits for malpractice have become increasingly frequent in recent years. The reasons are numerous and probably reflect the relatively lax medical staff discipline in many American hospitals, the increasing sophistication of patients, the aggressiveness of lawyers, the high costs of medical care (often not covered by insurance or in other ways), the tendency of insurance companies covering the doctor to settle claims of even dubious merit rather than run the risk of court litigation, the jury system even for noncriminal tort actions, and so on. In any event, the rate and amounts of malpractice awards or out-of-court financial settlements have risen so much that the personal liability insurance that nearly all American physicians carry has become extremely costly; premiums amount to many thousands of dollars a year, being especially high for surgeons and anesthesiologists. This malpractice crisis has led to intense protests, including strikes, by doctors and to many legislative reforms of the tort law in this field. At the same time, the patient's right to initiate such law suits has exerted an influence in heightening self-discipline within the medical care system, especially in hospitals.

Regulation of medical performance through the social insurance programs of the welfare state countries is somewhat more rigorous. The British general practitioner pattern with its capitation payment, for example, uses a simple approach: to protect quality, the government sets a maximum number of persons allowable on any GP list. In the more prevalent fee-for-service payment pattern, regulation is always more complicated. The German sickness funds conduct computerized reviews of each doctor's practice habits, as measured by such criteria as the number of drug prescriptions per case, number of office visits and laboratory tests per case, rates of certain surgical procedures, and so on. These measurements are compared with those of other doctors in the same specialty, and highly deviant individuals are readily identified. Such identification is regarded only as a screening step, to be followed up by detailed examination of the individual doctor's work. If this reveals unjustified services, the doctor may be penalized by payment of only a fraction of his claims; in seriously irregular instances, the doctor may be ruled out of participation in the social insurance program entirely.

In Canada, several of the provinces apply similar techniques for identifying doctors whose practice customs suggest abuse. Procedures are especially diligent in the province of Quebec, where the medical care insurance program transmits to the medical licensing body the names of doctors with deviant statistical profiles. The licensing body then calls on the doctor for an explanation, and if the explanation is not satisfactory, the penalty may be to require the doctor to undertake a certain course of postgraduate study or to have a second consultant in all subsequent cases of certain diagnoses. In general, these regulatory procedures probably exert more influence on the quality and costs of medical care by their mere existence than by the relatively few cases of irresponsible medical performance that they uncover.

Not every welfare state's health insurance system is equally rigorous in its regulatory practices. Belgium and Japan are examples of countries where the private medical profession is extremely powerful politically. Doctors have successfully resisted almost all efforts of the insurance program to discipline deviant behavior. In these countries, the social insurance program is regarded essentially as a payment mechanism that cannot challenge the decisions or performance of any licensed physician.

Professional societies in most of the welfare state countries generally fall into two types: (1) the association concerned with scientific advancement, including continuing education, and (2) the body concerned with negotiations on economic matters with government or social insurance organizations. The latter group also monitors the ethical behavior of its members. In addition, there are also various societies in the medical specialties, including general practice. In the nursing, pharmaceutical, and other health professions, these two distinct roles are sometimes played by committees or divisions of one national association. With the prevailing separation of general medical practitioners from hospitals in the welfare states, societies of GP's tend to have a great deal of vitality and are staunchly dedicated to advancement of the status of their members. As a result, they are particularly conscientious in promoting diligent performance.

For many reasons, the relative weights of which are not clear, legal actions for malpractice against doctors or hospitals or other providers of health services are quite rare in the welfare states. Most prominent among the causes is probably the national health insurance legislation, under which any medical costs due to malfeasance are covered, along with other health care costs. The more disciplined medical staff organization within hospitals (compared with that in the United States) also probably reduces poor performance. The legal systems concerning torts generally differ: contingency fees for lawyers are either prohibited or considered unethical, and jury trials are not used in civil (noncriminal) actions. Private insurance companies are not so commonly used for carrying malpractice liability insurance; instead, the medical associations often operate protective organizations to which all their members contribute premiums. Then, whenever the doctor's behavior has been considered reasonable, he is vigorously defended, rather than having financial settlement offered to avoid litigation. Finally, the effective personal relationships that tend to develop between patients and their general practitioners (who, it will be recalled, are proportionately much more numerous than in the United States) mean that patients seldom get angry with their doctors and the whole medical establishment. (In the United States, patient anger is the initial provocation of many law suits.) As a result, malpractice insurance premiums paid by doctors in Great Britain, Canada, Norway, and Australia average only about $100 a year—a trivial fraction of the rates in the United States.

In the developing countries, the organized health care programs usually pay doctors by salary, rather than by fees or capitation, so that the scheme of remuneration as such is not relied on for regulation of performance. Rather, it is the organizational dynamics within the delivery system—supervision, consultation, meritorious promotion, and so on—that influence the behavior of health care providers. As far as purely private professional practice is concerned, regulation is virtually nonexistent after professional licensure or registration.

Similarly, the professional societies do little if anything to discipline practitioners in the developing countries. The role of the societies is to educate their members on scientific advances and to negotiate with government and social insurance bodies on economic questions. In a sense, the diligence of medical and other societies in protecting patients against any malfeasance of health providers varies with the sophistication of the general population about scientific matters, which tends to be quite weak in the developing countries.

For the same reason, legal redress for patient grievances is seldom sought in the developing countries. Rare is the patient in Africa who would challenge the effects of a doctor's acts, or the lawyer who would represent him. Grievance procedures may sometimes operate in the social security medical care systems of the transitional countries, although these generally concern problems of accessibility (e.g., a long waiting time before seeing the doctor) rather than medical performance. A rather highly educated and sophisticated population is required to generate recourse to the courts for adjudicating the claims of patients about injuries resulting from improper medical care.

In the socialist countries, also, it is the structure of the entire delivery system that principally regulates the quality of medical care. The salaries paid to personnel and the responsibilities assigned to them embody rewards for competence, experience, and responsibility. Correspondingly, poor performance in the opinion of the organizational leadership may result in failure to advance, or even demotion. (In a way, the mechanism resembles that used in American universities, where the advancement of professors depends on the judgment of their colleagues and academic supervisors.) Thus, the scheme for payment of health personnel does, in fact, exercise an influence on performance by giving incentives through salary levels for diligent work. The judgment of merit, however, depends on professional peers rather than on popularity with patients.

Professional associations play only a very limited role in the socialist countries, outside the sphere of continuing education. Ethical constraints are exercised within the government health system itself. Since there is little if any private practice, however, the objective of opposing commercialized abuses, which generate most ethical codes in other societies, is not relevant. There are labor unions of health workers, including physicians, but their role is primarily to mediate grievances of personnel, to represent their members in salary negotiations, to conduct welfare programs (such as operating rest homes and vacation resorts), and so on.

Medical specialty societies in Poland, and probably in other socialist countries as well, play a semiofficial role in monitoring performance in their respective fields. Committees from each specialty body make periodic visits to all hospitals and polyclinics for monitoring the quality of the work in their particular fields. They give ratings on the quality of performance of individuals that influence the individuals' rates of promotion. If they find substandard performance, they may recommend transfer of certain personnel to another location where the individual's work will be more closely supervised. In addition, these committees may be summoned to consult on problems at a particular facility where the local medical director needs advice. An effort is made to include on these specialty committees doctors from both academic (or theoretical) and practical backgrounds of experience.

Judicial redress through the courts plays little part in the regulation of health care performance in socialist settings. A patient with cause for dissatisfaction or with an injury considered attributable to poor medical work brings his complaint to the attention of the supervisor of the program involved. If there are complaints from several persons, they might appeal to the political party machinery, which is intended to oversee the operations of all social programs. Courts of law, however, are confined largely to adjudication of criminal acts or alleged crimes. Even such matters as transfers of property, wills, business contracts, and the like, which occupy so much of the time of private lawyers in capitalist societies, are handled in socialist societies by government bureaus.

Thus, in all types of countries and in a variety of ways—governmental and voluntary—regulation over the health services has grown. While official licensure of health personnel has been the fundamental approach, various forms of approval or control have been applied increasingly to other kinds of health resources, such as facilities and drugs. Regulation of the day-to-day performance of health services has been extended through diverse methods of surveillance or teamwork patterns for organizing health care delivery. As the financing of health care by the whole population becomes more collectivized, pressures mount for greater regulation to control both the costs and quality of services.

Readings

Altenstetter, Christa, *Health Policy-Making and Administration in West Germany and the United States*, Beverly Hills, Calif.: Sage Publications, 1974.

Beck, R. G., "The Effects of Co-Payment on the Poor," *Journal of Human Resources*, 9:129-141 (Winter 1974).

Bridgman, Robert F. and Milton I. Roemer, *Hospital Legislation and Hospital Systems*, Geneva: World Health Organization, Public Health Papers No. 50, 1973.

Curran, W. J., "Legan Regulation and Quality Control of Medical Practice under the National Health Service," *New England Journal of Medicine, 274*:547 (March 1966).

Dunlop, D. M., "Drug Control and the British Health Service," *Annals of Internal Medicine, 71*:237-244 (1969).

Dussault, René, "Quebec's Professional Code Requires Radical Restructure of Professional Organization," *Canadian Medical Association Journal, 111*: 724 (October 1974).

Fry, John, "Regulation and Control of the Medical Profession in Great Britain," *International Journal of Health Services, 6*:5-8 (1976).

Hansen, Horace R., *Medical Licensure and Consumer Protection: An Analysis and Evaluation of State Medical Licensure*, Washington, D.C.: Group Health Association of America, 1962.

Hill, Lawrence A., "Hospital Costs and Controls in Canada and the United States," *Health Services Research, 4*:170-176 (1969).

Krause, Elliott A., "The Political Context of Health Service Regulation," *International Journal of Health Services, 5*:593-608 (1975).

Laframboise, H. L. and T. H. Owen, "Surveillance Methodology for the Practice of Medicine," *Canadian Medical Association Journal, 106*:593-598 (March 1972).

Lewin and Associates, *Government Controls on the Health Care System: The Canadian Experience*, Washington, D.C.: 1976.

Roemer, Milton I., "Social Insurance as Leverage for Changing Health Care Systems: International Experience," *Bulletin of the New York Academy of Medicine, 48* (January 1972).

———, "The Expanding Scope of Governmental Regulation of Health Care Delivery," *University of Toledo Law Review, 6*:591-616 (Spring 1975).

Roemer, Ruth, "Abortion Law' The Approaches of Different Nations," *American Journal of Public Health, 57*:1906-1922 (November 1967).

———, "Legal Systems Regulating Health Personnel: A Comparative Analysis," *Milbank Memorial Fund Quarterly, 46*:431-471 (October 1968).

Shryock, Richard L., *Medical Licensing in America 1650-1965*, Baltimore: Johns Hopkins Press, 1967.

Sigerist, Henry E., "The History of Medical Licensure," *Journal of the American Medical Association, 104*:1056-1060 (March 1935).

Silverstein, Arthur, "Liability of the Physician in Jewish Law," *Israel Law Review, 10*:378 (1975).

Snyder, Francis, G., "Health Policy and the Law in Senegal," *Social Science and Medicine, 8*:11-28 (January 1974).

Somers, Anne R., *Hospital Regulation: The Dilemma of Public Policy,* Princeton, N. J.: Princeton University, Industrial Relations Section, 1969.

Speller, S. R., *Law Relating to Hospitals and Kindred Institutions,* 4th ed., London: Lewis, 1965.

Stevens, Rosemary, *Medical Practice in Modern England: The Impact of Specialization and State Medicine,* New Haven: Yale University Press, 1966.

Thorsen, Laurence C., "How Can the U.S. Government Control Physicians' Fees under National Health Insurance? A Lesson from the French System," *International Journal of Health Services, 4*:49-57 (1974).

U.S. Department of Health, Education, & Welfare, *Report of the Secretary's Commission of Medical Malpractice,* Washington, D.C.: Government Printing Office, January 1973.

World Health Organization, "Specialization: A Survey of Existing Legislation," *International Digest of Health Legislation, 8*:561 (1957).

World Health Organization, *Distribution and Trade in Pharmaceutical Preparations: A Survey of Existing Legislation,* Geneva, WHO, 1962.

World Health Organization, *Auxiliary Personnel in Nursing: A Survey of Existing Legislation,* Geneva, WHO, 1966.

World Health Organization, *Equivalence of Medical Qualifications and the Practice of Medicine: A Survey of Existing Legislation,* Geneva: WHO, 1967.

Worthington, William and Laurens H. Silver, "Regulation of Quality of Care in Hospitals: The Need for Change," *Law and Contemporary Problems, 35*: 305-333 (Spring 1970).

9

HEALTH SERVICE ADMINISTRATION AND PLANNING

In modern societies, health service systems do not just run themselves automatically. Beyond regulation, considered in the previous chapter, the dynamics of a system require some form of administration or management. With varying degrees of deliberate intent, priorities are formulated and planning is done to prepare for the future.

This chapter will examine the general administrative structure of the health service system in different types of countries, including the balance between centralized and decentralized authority, the relationships between political and technical considerations, governmental and voluntary responsibilities, the place of consumers, and problems of coordination. Next we will look at the different forms of social planning used to achieve certain goals along dimensions of economic support, output of resources (manpower and facilities), and the shaping of health care delivery patterns. Finally, we will consider the variations in decisions on health priorities made in the light of competing demands for resources in different types of countries; here we may see the trends appearing around the world toward achievement of health service equity. The blending of politics and health care systems is implicit in every aspect of those systems, but in the health administration and planning dynamics of countries this connection is dramatically prominent for everyone to see.

Administrative Structure

In the earliest societies, when the totality of health service consisted of individual healer-patient relationships, there was no need for systematic administration. However, as soon as groups of people became involved in the economic support or the organization of any type of health service, some mechanism became necessary for the exercise of authority. As nations have taken shape, authority has been exercised with differing balances between centralization and local autonomy or the peripheral delegation of power. Within governments, decisions involve various blends of political and technical considerations. Furthermore, government has various degrees of responsibility in relation to private or voluntary entities. Since health service involves interrelationships between providers and patients or consumers, there may be various levels of participation of each party in the exercise of authority. And as multiple organized health programs come into operation, problems of articulation arise between and among them. Different methods of coordination have been developed to keep the system as a whole operating effectively.

Free Enterprise Systems

In the free enterprise setting, the theme for the exercise of authority has been maximum possible decentralization. The United States were founded from a revolution against centralized power, and the constitutional structure of the nation defines a federation of semiautonomous states. Health service is one of many functions for which the state governments are primarily responsible. Similar federations of states or provinces are found in other countries, such as Australia or Canada, that, until recently, would have been characterized as free enterprise in type. Insofar as government exercises controls over the financing, delivery, quality, or other aspects of health service, it is mainly at the state or provincial level, or even more locally at the county or municipal level to which the state or provincial government may delegate certain responsibilities.

As health service has come to require increased economic support from public revenues and as taxing powers in our intermeshed economy have become relatively greater at the federal level, the national government has come to play a larger role. This has been done in large part through federal grants to the states, with various conditions for those grants being stipulated. In recent decades, moreover, the U.S. Supreme Court has interpreted the Constitution to allow somewhat greater direct federal authority under its general welfare clause. Thus, for example a federal social security tax is now used to finance medical care for aged pensioners (Medicare). In the administration of even this program, however, agencies of the state government and even voluntary bodies defined by state borders are directly involved. Responsibilities for many more components of health service rest squarely within the states.

With increased communication and democratization of American society, nevertheless, a sense of national identity has replaced much local or state identity, which has resulted in demands for greater uniformity in health care throughout the nation. In practical terms, these demands have led increasingly to national standards, even though the implementation of most health programs may rest with the states. To compensate for the variable economic levels among the states, federal grants may be issued on a variable matching basis, so that the poorer states receive greater proportions of federal support. The redistributional effect of such a policy enables the states to achieve or at least approach uniform quality of services. Sometimes national standards are issued for purely voluntary guidance, such as those issued by the U.S. Public Health Service for the handling of milk or those issued by the American Public Health Association, a voluntary body, for the immunization of children.

In the United States, as indeed in nearly all countries, the highest health officials in both national and state governments are determined by political more than technical considerations. They are, however, typically appointed rather than elected. A state director of public health or the members of a state medical licensing board are usually appointed by the state governor. Similarly at the federal level, the Secretary of the Department of Health, Education and Welfare, which contains the U.S. Public Health Service and other important agencies, is appointed by the president. These officials are not members of the elected federal Congress, and they are usually expected to have some technical competence, but their selection depends mainly on political or ideological criteria.

Just as responsibilities for health service rest with local more than centralized authorities, they are carried more by private or voluntary than by governmental bodies in the free enterprise setting. We have already noted that most general hospital beds in the United States are in voluntary institutions and most physicians are in private practice. A great deal of government money for health purposes is spent through the purchase of services from these private providers. Private universities and colleges are heavily supported by government grants, just as medical research, although it is conducted by scientists in both private and state government institutions, is financed mainly by federal grants. When a nation as large as the United States has no national department of health at the level of the president's cabinet but, rather, combines health with several other public responsibilities, one may infer the weakness of health service in the government domain as compared to the private.

The very strength of the private forces, which are largely dominated by the providers of care, has given rise in the United States to a mounting demand for greater participation of patients or consumers in the management of the health services. In the last decade, this trend has mainly taken the form of demands by ethnic minority groups who have suffered special disadvantages in our free enterprise health care system. However, the basic issue of consumer control has also been expressed in many other forms for many years. The control of hospitals, both voluntary and public, has long been predominantly by the consumers of their services, although the consumers seldom represent the general population.

Some health insurance plans are sponsored by consumers, although it is noteworthy that the largest ones in America are sponsored by commercial companies
or by the providers of hospital (Blue Cross) or medical (Blue Shield) services.
An increasing number of administrative boards required under new United States
health legislation must be composed of a majority of consumers.

The very multiplicity of American health agencies, both public and private,
has created special problems of coordination. In the realm of government, there
are periodic reorganizations for the purpose of achieving greater efficiency. One
of the common steps at the local level in recent years has been to amalgamate
previously separate departments of public health, government hospitals, and
mental health. At local, state, and national levels, one sees numerous nonofficial
health councils bringing together representatives of diverse private and public
agencies. The hospitals in a region may join together in a special hospital council
to coordinate their efforts; agencies in specialized fields, such as mental health
care, chronic disease control, or child health, may likewise come together to
avoid duplication of efforts and identify program gaps. The complexity of
agencies and programs in the United States has stimulated increased interest in
comprehensive health planning, which will be discussed later.

Welfare State Systems

The administrative structure of health services in the welfare states is different
in many ways. On the whole, the position of government is much stronger,
usually at a central rather than local level. In welfare states there are many variations, some putting greater stress for certain functions on local health authority
than others. In Norway, for example, the control of hospitals is vested largely
in local county governments, although most of their financial support comes
from a social insurance law that is nationally operated. British hospitals, on the
other hand, are nominally controlled by the central government, but their daily
administration is delegated to local representatives appointed by the national
minister. Most French general hospitals are owned and operated by the *département,* but they must follow rules established by the central authorities.

Much more than in the United States, the welfare states follow national
health policies, even when day-to-day administration is decentralized. The same
recent trends toward increasingly centralized powers that we have described for
the United States have been occurring in Western Europe and at a greater pace,
as is well illustrated in the health insurance programs that generally started with
the operation of numerous autonomous local sickness funds. Much of the initial
social insurance legislation in Europe simply mandated enrollment of people in
a local society. Then gradually the laws were amended, so that in many countries
the local funds became, in effect, branches of an integrated national network of

agencies. The collection of insurance taxes became centralized, and monies were then allocated to the local units for payment or reimbursement for the services rendered. Belgium, with its hundreds of still autonomous benefit societies, is an exception to this trend, but the general Western European structure of health services embodies largely centralized authority.

Even the nominations of hospital doctors are made by the central government in Norway and Sweden, although the local authorities do the appointing. Similarly, the country-wide network of district doctors in Norway depends on central ministry selection and supervision. Sanitation codes are national, and educational institutions are generally approved by the central Ministry of Education. Of course, the European countries are smaller than the United States, both in area and population, but Great Britain has 55,000,000 people, which is much more than Canada or Australia with their federated patterns. On the other hand, Switzerland with under 5,000,000 population is a federation of twenty four separate cantons, each of which, unlike patterns in the rest of Europe, has great autonomy in health affairs, as in almost everything else. In Switzerland as in Belgium, it is history rather than size that explains the deviation from general welfare state administrative patterns.

The electoral process in Europe is much more important than technical factors in the designation of top health authorities. Under the parliamentary government system, a minister of health is chosen by the majority party from the members of the parliament, each of whom has been elected by some local district. It is rare, therefore, to have a medical doctor as health minister. Aneurin Bevan, whose leadership launched the British National Health Service, was a former coal miner. Under the minister is a chief medical officer, a director-general of health services, or the like—a person selected by the minister for his technical competence, although he also usually reflects a compatible viewpoint. The boards governing local government hospitals may also be elected or may be appointed by elected officials.

Many of the welfare state insurance organizations are politically oriented. There are often certain funds whose leadership comes from the Christian Democrats, others from the Socialists, others that are deliberately neutral, and so on. Since political activities representing organized workers or other social classes have long been in great ferment in Western Europe, there are usually numerous political parties that may form coalitions, in contrast to the two-party system of the United States. In coalition governments, the major ministries, such as foreign affairs, finance, or military defense, usually go to the major parties, and relatively secondary ministries, including health or labor affairs, go to the minor political parties. Thus, in the French coalition government following World War II, the Labor Ministry was assigned to a member of the Communist Party, and it was at this time that France enacted its especially comprehensive program for the health protection of industrial workers.

In the health administrative structure, government agencies in most welfare state countries tend to be more important than voluntary agencies. The distinction between these two types, moreover, is not so sharp. Thus, the separation between church and state, so fundamental in the United States, is not found in Western Europe. Many European countries have an official national church, the acitivites of which—including schools and hospitals—are supported by public revenues. Voluntary health agencies are generally well subsidized by government; their objectives are more to mobilize the efforts of private citizens for various health purposes than to raise money. Competition between voluntary and public agencies, observed often in the United States, is seldom seen in the welfare states.

The issue of consumerism—so prominent in the American health scene in recent years—is not significant in the welfare states. Perhaps this is because, through the political process and the general administrative structure of the health services, consumers have long played a major role. In contrast to consumers in the United States, they dominate the health insurance movement, the public health authorities, and the hospital boards whose members are more likely to be representative of the general population than of wealthy donors. Hence, the sense of powerlessness, which stimulated the consumer movement in American health services, has not been felt in Western Europe.

Problems of coordination among health agencies exist in the welfare states, although to a lesser degree than in the free enterprise setting. The major issue is within the sphere of government, in the relationships between ministries of health and other ministries (often labor or social welfare) responsible for the health insurance and social security systems. The many coordinating councils, generated by the vast multiplicity of public and private health agencies in the United States, are not seen so often in the Western European countries.

Developing Country Systems

Health administrative structures in both the transitional and underdeveloped countries, especially in the latter, are usually still more centralized than in the welfare states. Local government in these countries, where general levels of education are rather low, is typically weak. Authority, therefore, is usually exercised by central governments. If there are provinces or other regional jurisdictions, their governmental officials are usually appointed by the central power rather than being locally elected. In Egypt and Ecuador, for example, almost every administrative decision in a governmental hospital or health center must be approved at the top level. This may apply to the purchase of almost any sort of supply or the appointment of even the humblest employee. Efforts are being made in some countries to decentralize decision making—often through centrally appointed regional officials to whom many responsibilities are delegated—but such efforts are slow. Even after being appointed, regional health directors often hesitate to make decisions on their own for fear that they might cause dissatisfaction at higher levels and jeopardize their appointments.

As between political and technical considerations, there is no question about the great preeminence of the former in health policy decisions of developing countries. A great many governments in Latin America and Africa are the result of military coups rather than general elections, and the ministers of health are often officers of the armed forces. Decisions on health affairs are largely motivated by political rather than objective technical criteria. For example, large monumental hospitals in the capital city, intended to impress people with the grandeur of the central government, are often constructed with funds that might have built dozens of small rural health centers. In part, such decisions are also made to impress foreign dignitaries, whose visits are generally confined to the national capital.

Another reflection of political rather than technical criteria is seen in the appointments of public officials in the developing countries. True merit systems are rare, and nepotism is common. Relatives are appointed not only because of the personal economic advantages of government appointments but also because they are considered politically trustworthy. A health service administrator, appointed solely on the basis of technical qualifications, might well make decisions contrary to the policies of the top executive in the health system. A frequent by-product of such tendencies is the frustration of young public health doctors sent overseas for technical training; when they return home after schooling, the national rulers have often changed. As a result, the position for which their training was intended has meanwhile been filled with someone else. Anticipating this, many health personnel from developing countries sent abroad for graduate studies do not return home.

In the developing countries generally, voluntary agencies are relatively unimportant. Government is much more influential, and often voluntary bodies formed mainly for reasons of political expedience soon become dependent on government for economic support. Family planning agencies, discussed earlier, illustrate this, and their support may come from foreign governments as well as their own. Religious missions are also largely dependent on foreign support, although it is not government support. The church-sponsored hospitals of Latin America are not only financed largely by government but have come increasingly under government control.

There is little consumer participation in the administration of the health care systems of developing countries, nor is there very much demand for such a role. Pressures for representation of the average person on decision-making bodies depend on high levels of education and political consciousness, which are seldom found in the less developed countries. Yet some governments, such as that of Tanzania or Panama, may deliberately encourage village councils to play an administrative role in health service administration. Such policies are doubtless growing, but in most developing countries they arise more from the initiative of the central governments themselves than from demand at the grass roots level.

In the severely underdeveloped countries, coordination among health agencies is not a serious problem because there are not so many different organizations involved. In the transitional countries with social security health programs, however, there have arisen serious rivalries with ministries of health. Since the social security bodies have a separate source of funds, they make decisions on their use independently. Various committees have been appointed to coordinate efforts, and joint use of certain hospitals by both agencies has often been arranged to avoid wasteful duplication. With the Chilean National Health Service of 1952, full integration of the social security and ministry of health programs, as well as the *beneficencia* hospitals, was achieved. More recently in Costa Rica, all personal health services in both hospitals and health centers were integrated under the social security authorities. However, in most transitional countries, the separation of various health care programs remains a problem.

Socialist Systems

In the socialist countries, the administrative structure of the health services has become basically simplified. Following the example of the Soviet Union, policies on virtually every aspect of health service are formulated by the central ministry of health. Goals are specified and standards are set, with implementation delegated peripherally through a pyramidal network of authorities. Although budgets are prepared at the local level and sent in, through steps, to the central government, nearly all funds for health program operation are allocated outwardly by the central body. The administrative pattern in the People's Republic of China is much more decentralized. Although general health policies are promulgated from the center through the political party organization, their implementation depends very largely on the initiative of local authorities, mainly through the rural communes. Financial support is provided from the resources and productivity at the several levels—provinces, counties, and communes or municipalities, as well as partly from the central government. As a result, there are much greater differences in the standards of health service attainable in different regions of this large country than are found in the Soviet Union. Local self-reliance is an important principle in China that is applied to health service as well as to agriculture, housing, and other aspects of life.

Political judgments prevail over technical judgments in all the socialist health systems. Perhaps it is this very fact that has led these countries to put so high a priority on building up the resources for health care, since this has been a way to win the support of the people as well as to heighten the productivity of the economy. There are no parliamentary elections in the usual sense in these countries, but within the Communist Party structure there are votes and debates among the spokesmen for contending viewpoints. Top health officials at each government level are selected by the Communist Party organization, and their choice is based more on their political trustworthiness than on their technical competence. In the Soviet Union, there has been some evidence of increasing influence by the specialized experts in various fields. It was partly in reaction to such "technocratic" and "bureaucratic" tendencies in China that the Proletarian Cultural Revolution broke out in 1966-1969 and resulted in a reaffirmation of the primacy of the "masses," as against the "experts."

Government, rather than private entities, is obviously all-important in the socialist health systems. Yet voluntary agencies still exist to a small degree. There are Red Cross or equivalent societies for giving aid in emergencies, and much of their service is contributed by unpaid volunteers. In Cuba, a network of nongovernment Committees for the Defense of the Revolution (CDR) has been organized under the stimulus of the ruling political party. The CDRs assist on a volunteer basis in various health campaigns, such as cleaning up city streets or persuading mothers to bring their children to the health centers for immunizations.

According to the ideology of the socialist countries, the Communist Party represents the mass of the population, so that there is no need for any separate consumerism movement. Although many would be skeptical of this judgment, the Party organization itself serves as a kind of grievance channel through which patients may bring complaints about the operation of the health services. Any significant grievances, either expressed or observable, may induce the local Party unit to initiate corrective actions.

With respect to coordination of health services, the problems are minimal in the socialist frameworks. Whatever may be lacking in personal freedom, the systems are manifestly unified and integrated. "Socialist competition" is promoted between localities—for example, in achieving low infant mortality rates or high rates of "dispensarization" of the population—but competitive duplication of resources or efforts is minimal.

Health Service Planning

Planning in health services, as in many other sectors of society, has had many different meanings. In a sense, any systematic course of action in which sequential steps are contemplated constitutes planning. Every individual plans his or her day with various degrees of rigor, and every organization plans its program with various degrees of thoroughness and detail. The variations in the geographic scope of a plan may be enormous, ranging from a particular business enterprise or a small village all the way up to a whole nation or even to the entire world.

In health services, the application of planning has naturally reflected the ideology of the whole nation. Every hospital, every doctor's practice, every nurse's day involves planning, but by common consent health service planning has come to mean the systematic approach to the production and use of resources that is advocated by the national government. This does not mean that all planning is done solely in the nation's capital but, rather, that in the national government there is a concept of planning that may be carried out entirely there or at different political levels throughout the land. A nation's concept of planning may delegate decision-making responsibilities to a few large regions, to numerous provinces, or even to hundreds of local communities. However, in the nation's political headquarters there is a certain concept that, as we shall see, differs substantially among the different types of country.

The very idea of planning at a central level has been most deliberately formulated in the socialist nations. Contrary to our practice in previous chapters, therefore, we will begin our review with those systems and conclude with the free enterprise system. We must not forget, however, that almost every *organized* health action taken either by government or by a voluntary body at any level since ancient times has constituted a type of health planning. Whenever a hospital was built, when a barber-surgeon's guild was formed or a professional licensure law was passed, when a cancer society was founded, when a medical fee schedule was issued, when a health insurance plan was organized, when a program for helping crippled children was established—all these constituted a form of health care planning. Within the meaning of this chapter, nevertheless, it may be most helpful to consider planning as *intervention in the free market for production or distribution of health services.* The most extensive intervention of this sort was undertaken in the Soviet Union after the Russian Revolution, and it has gradually spread with varying impact throughout the world.

Socialist Systems

The early days after the first socialist revolution in Russia in 1918 were very turbulent, and the energies of the ruling majority Bolshevik Party were directed for several years to establishing a framework of government and to consolidating power. It was not until 1928, ten years after the Revolution, that enough stability was achieved to prepare the first Five Year Plan—a concept, incidentally, not envisaged by Marx or Engels. Planning came to mean the consideration of the total economic and social scene, with deliberate stipulation of goals deemed reachable by collective action in a certain period of time; movement had to be expected along several paths simultaneously, and health care was, of course, only one among many. Since health care required, for example, the construction of hospitals and health centers, there had to be concurrent progress in the construction industry, which depended in turn on production of steel and cement, and so on. There also had to be concurrent actions to train health personnel and to pay them—hence, the organization of a flow of money through tax collection (social insurance and general revenue) systems, and then mechanisms for setting and distributing salaries.

Without reviewing all the elaborate steps involved, the socialist pattern of health planning today is highly centralized, although its implementation natuarlly depends on thousands of local actions. In the central government is a principal planning body for the total society, known by a Russian acronyn as GOSPLAN. In each ministry, formerly called *commissariats*, there is also a planning body responsible for the more detailed course of action within the broad framework of goals stipulated by GOSPLAN. In the Health Ministry, the planning is done primarily at a sort of research organization known as the Semashko Institute (named after the Soviet Union's first Minister of Health and a participant, with Lenin, in the 1918 Revolution).

The Semashko Institute is devoted primarily to the formulation of health goals deemed attainable within the constraints of (1) the monies allocated by GOSPLAN to the health sector, and (2) the circumstances and competing pressures expected over a five-year period. The exact techniques followed in defining these goals have naturally changed over the last fifty years, but today they are expressed largely in terms of standards or norms that are to be attained in all subdivisions of the health service. At first, these norms were used simply to achieve some quantitative improvements over the obviously deficient levels of resources and services originally available to the people. For example, just before the Revolution there were about 21,000 physicians in Russia or, for its population then (about 125,000,000), a ratio of approximately 1:6,000. This was obviously inadequate, and the new government set out immediately to train many more doctors by setting up medical schools in all the main cities. By the end of the first decade (1928), the number of doctors had been tripled to 63,000. After the first Five Year Plan, the number of doctors had been further increased to over 76,000, or a ratio of about 1:2,000. As experience was gained, health planning was carried out on a more refined basis, with more accurate measurements of needs. The strategy that eventually developed may be described as a combination of empiricism, theory, and social value judgments.

Thus, today empirical estimates on the *need* for physicians, as well as all other types of health manpower, facilities, and equipment are made initially through measurements of the demands for medical care—all of which is free or offered as a public service—actually expressed in selected experimental communities of different types. These types are: (1) the small village or rural area, (2) the middle-sized town, and (3) the average neighborhood of a large city. It is realized that levels of transportation, education, and also attitudes toward health differ in these three types of environment. The basic setting at which demands are quantified is the polyclinic or health center that serves a district of known population. At these experimental units, a generous supply of health manpower is provided so that the population's demands for health care may be expressed with virutally no constraints, such as long waiting periods (which might discourage seeking care in the first place).

The doctors and allied personnel at the study units are expected and instructed to give the patients all the care they need. If someone requires hospitalization, he or she is to be referred for it. Likewise, a general practitioner (therapeutist), who is always seen first, refers the patient to a specialist when it is deemed necessary. Diagnostic tests are performed, drugs are prescribed, and so on, according to the doctor's judgment. General social policy in the USSR has established that the doctor's average work day should be six hours, shorter than for most workers, since the tasks of medicine are considered to be especially stressful. Then, if more doctors are found necessary to meet the demand at the polyclinic without there being excessive waiting time, they are engaged. On this basis, the number of consultations for physicians' care in each type of setting is tabulated and, considering the total population served, a rate of services per 1,000 persons per year is calculated.

These empirical rates are then studied in the light of various theoretical factors. One such factor is the presence of illness for which care has not been sought. Data on this factor are obtained by medical examination surveys of entire populations, sick and well. Another factor is the theoretical need for preventive services, including health education, for which people would not ordinarily seek service without aggressive publicity or outreach efforts. On the basis of such theoretical factors, the empirical rates estimated as above are modified by committees of experts.

Finally, judgments are made on the working efficiency of the doctors and other health personnel. Did some work too slowly and others too hastily? Such judgments are obviously value judgments made according to the prevailing knowledge of the time and prevailing conceptions of good medical care. After tabulating the average number of patients (including initial visits, which may be lengthy, and more brief revisits) actually seen per hour by generalists and different specialists, an ideal standard is stipulated. Recently, the standard was five patients per hour for general practitioners, for example. Allowance must also be made for time spent by the doctor on home calls during the six-hour working day.

On the basis of these three forms of measurement, a standard or norm is calculated on the number of physicians of each specialty required per 10,000 population in a community of the stated type. Through comparable determination of the rate of cases hospitalized and their durations of stay, the numbers of hospital beds required are calculated and distributed among institutions of different sizes and levels of technical complexity according to a regionalization pattern. All these measurements, tabulations, and calculations are repeated every few years to make adjustments for changes in medical science, in disease patterns, in educational levels and attitudes of people, in transportation facilities, in the use and availability of allied health personnel, in concepts of disease prevention or health promotion, and so on.

The norms so computed are then applied in planning the output of the nation's medical schools, the specialty preparation programs, and so on. They are also used for the preparation and review of personnel establishments and budgets to support health care programs in villages, towns, and cities of the three types. Thus, in 1970 there was a net supply of 668,400 doctors in the Soviet Union (this does not count the middle-level *feldsher,* but it does include the stomatologist) or about 1:362. The plan for 1975 called for 830,000 doctors or a ratio of about 1:308 population, much more than in any other nation. It must, however, be kept in mind that the Soviet doctor's working day is shorter than that in most other countries, so that the aggregate medical time available is not quite as much as these ratios might suggest.

Equivalent combinations of empiricism, theoretical estimates of need, and social value judgments are applied to the planning of all elements in the Soviet health care system. Since the achievement of goals in the health sector each five years obviously depends on balanced planning in other sectors (e.g., in the chemical industry for manufacture of drugs, in agriculture for the feeding of hospital patients, etc.), the entire process requires highly sophisticated coordination at the central level of GOSPLAN. Mistakes in calculations are naturally made, and goals in certain fields may not be reached (e.g., agriculture has fallen behind in the production of many foodstuffs, necessitating large imports) so that shortcomings in one sector may affect the achievement of goals in other sectors. Serious disruptions in the whole planning process may also be caused by wars, natural catastrophies, or civil disruptions. Nevertheless, the entire process is clearly intended to map out a rational production of resources and services proportionate to the estimated health needs within the constraints present at each time and place. The delivery of health services is based on a centrally planned determination of needs, with virtually no influence from a free market of individual demands, supply, and price.

This somewhat oversimplified account of the Soviet model of health care planning is essentially emulated, with varying modifications, by most but not all other socialist countries. In Yugoslavia, we know that there is much greater decentralization of decision making to the six provinces (republics) of that country. In each province, however, a somewhat similar process is carried out, although the over-all allocation of funds to the health sector, compared with other needs, appears to be less than in the USSR. In the People's Republic of China, much of the health planning is also far more decentralized to the provinces (twenty five) and counties (2,000), although certain system components—such as the output of physicians and of barefoot doctors—appear to be centrally determined.

In many ways, the concept of planning pioneered by the Soviet Union has also been emulated by other nonsocialist countries, although to a much lesser degree and scope. In the health services and in education, perhaps, this highly rational model of planning has been applied more extensively than in many other sectors of society, where the freedom of the natural market is supported by stronger political interests.

Underdeveloped Countries

Looking to African nations as representing the underdeveloped country systems of health care, we find that virtually all of them are engaged in some form of centralized planning of health services. In general, there is an over-all planning program in the office of the president or prime minister, within which one section is devoted to health services. In addition, there is usually some unit in the ministry of health, or its equivalent, that is also devoted to planning and maintaining some sort of liaison with the generalized planning body. Sometimes the scope of the health ministry's planning responsibilities may be limited to one element, such as health centers. Health manpower planning, moreover, may be lodged mainly with the ministry of education.

Although the intent may be highly rational, the achievements of health planning in most of Africa have been quite limited. At this stage of history, the resources of these countries are extremely lean and, even with hard work, the goals must usually be very modest. With this is linked the crucial fact that in none of the African countries, as of this writing, has a broad egalitarian philosophy been implemented. There continues to exist everywhere a substantial private market sector in which health services are distributed on the basis of individual purchasing power. There are a few countries, such as Guinea, Tanzania, or Angola, where a democratic or semisocialist philosophy seems to be growing, but even in these, the sector of private ownership and distribution is still substantial. Thus, whatever planning is done is, in large measure, fractional; that is, it is limited to the public sector.

Accordingly, in Ghana, Nigeria, Kenya, Ethiopia, and most sub-Sahara African countries, one finds national health plans that call for construction of public hospitals and health centers at central government expense according to a regionalization concept. These hospitals are to be staffed with a few doctors but principally with allied health personnel, including the doctor-substitute variety. Primary care, both preventive and therapeutic, is intended to be available from health assistants in the rural villages, either without charge or for very small fees. Ambulance transportation is supposed to be associated with all the hospitals, and the health centers may be expected to dispatch mobile clinics to cover the distant villages. There are also plans for public water systems (usually community wells with pumps, rather than plumbing in houses), sewerage networks in the cities, latrines for rural households, and other measures of environmental sanitation. Campaigns for vector control to reduce parasitic and other communicable diseases are likewise in the national health plans.

In practice, however, all too often the plans remain largely on paper. Some hospitals may be built in the main African cities, but the schedule for construction of rural health centers typically fails to be attained. Even when construction of facilities is completed, the staffing seldom reaches the level intended. Training programs rarely turn out the numbers of skilled health personnel required. The most critical shortage generally applies to doctors. Those doctors who are trained in the country or overseas become engaged predominantly in private practice in the main cities, and the government medical posts are difficult to fill. Salaries in the government posts are relatively low, so that when a position is filled by a doctor, he is usually free also to engage in private practice to supplement his income, with the result that the public work seldom gets his full devotion.

A partial exception to this generally bleak picture of health planning and achievement is seen in Tanzania. As far back as 1938, a network of health centers was advocated in the British colony, then called Tanganyika, but the first one was established only in 1952. A five-year plan was drawn up in 1956 calling for forty health centers, each to serve about 50,000 people. By 1961, however, only twenty two had been put in operation, and forty were not set up until 1965. Then, in 1967 a new policy was laid down by the governing Tanganyika African National Union (TANU) Party. Known as the Arusha Declaration, this policy called for giving priority to the rural areas, with a great increase in the pace of establishing rural health centers and simple dispensaries. By 1973, there were 108 health centers in operation and over 1,500 small dispensaries. Indicative of the modesty of the plans is the staffing of both health centers and dispensaries by only medical assistants, nurses, and aides. The health centers have a few beds for maternity cases or emergencies, but physicians are planned for and located only in the hospitals.

At the most local level, in the smallest Tanzanian villages, the planning since 1967 has called for simple health posts, staffed by village medical helpers who are given three to six months training at a district hospital and are taught to treat minor ailments, provide first aid for more serious conditions, and offer preventive services. More thoroughly trained is the rural medical aide, who studies for three years after primary school (seven years). These personnel, who treat the majority of disorders, staff the dispensaries and most of the health centers. They are intended as true doctor substitutes. An even higher level of health worker is the licensed medical practitioner, who has had ten years of primary and secondary school, three years of health training, followed by four years of experience and then eighteen months of up-grading. Since there were in 1973 only 530 doctors in Tanzania (230 Tanzanian and 300 foreign), or a ratio of about 1:23,000 for the 14 million population, one can understand the planning for large numbers of allied health personnel. A major aspect of the rural development effort in Tanzania has been to promote cooperative or *ujamaa* villages in which local self-reliance and a collective spirit, inspired by the People's Republic of China, are emphasized.

Transitional Countries

Compared with most of Africa, India is a transitional country, at least as far as its health care system is concerned. Since 1951, a series of five-year plans have been launched that encompass all aspects of society, including health. Although the broad lines for health planning have been drawn at the national level, the execution of the health plans is left mainly to the sixteen federated states (plus eight centrally administered territories).

Under the state governments, health planning has called for the establishment and staffing of pyramidal networks of hospitals, health centers, and peripheral health stations, staffed principally by full-time state government personnel. The health center is the key facility for delivering ambulatory care, preventive and therapeutic, to a population of 80,000 to 100,000. Each unit is supposed to be staffed by at least one full-time physician and about forty other allied personnel. Approximately 5,500 of these facilities have so far been established under the successive five-year plans. Linked to each main health center are supposed to be several subcenters for every 10,000 people, staffed only by auxiliary personnel, but most of those needed have not yet been built. At the health centers, the planning calls also for services of sanitation workers and health education personnel.

Partly through these state-operated facilities and partly through separate units, the central government of India operates vertical programs for population control (family planning) and campaigns to attack tuberculosis, smallpox, malaria, and leprosy. Federal government grants are also made to the states for designated health purposes. Serious problems of poor coordination between central and state government activities have characterized planning in India, as emphasized in the major study of the Health Survey and Planning Committee (the Mudaliar Report) of 1961. Since then, other emphases of the five-year plans have been the construction of public water systems and the energetic promotion of birth control through a variety of methods. India's high birth rate, however, has been only slightly reduced, since effective family planning evidently depends much more on the level of general education and motivation of the people than on the availability of contraceptive techniques.

Perhaps equally important in the failure of India to achieve the goals of its several five-year plans for health has been the permissive ideology of the government with respect to private medical and hospital care. In spite of the enormous gaps in the health services of the state and central governments, only about 40 percent of the doctors trained are employed in the public programs, on which about 90 percent of the people depend along with their use of traditional healers. The other 60 percent of scientifically trained physicians engage in private medical practice in the larger cities, or they emigrate to other countries. Even greater public-private disparities apply to dental, pharmaceutical, and vision-care services. The ruling Congress Party of India is, in large part, controlled by mercantile interests that do not seem to wish to intervene in the private medical market.

In Latin America we see somewhat similar problems in planning—namely, a fractional approach directed only to the segment of resources that is within the public sector. In contrast to India, however (with its tradition of full-time employment of doctors in the colonial Indian Medical Service), most Latin American countries operate subsystems of health care that engage doctors for two, four, or six hours per day, the balance of their time being devoted to private practice. Hence, a much higher percentage of doctors, about 80 or 90 percent, work on part-time salaries in some organized program, but about 50 percent of their aggregate hours of work is devoted to private patients. As in India, therefore, this substantial private sector reduces the impact of health planning.

Important also in Latin America is the formulation of manpower and facility development plans, not only by the ministries of health and the health sections of over-all planning agencies, but also by the separate social security programs providing health care. There may be still other health plans made by voluntary agencies or by other special branches of the government. As noted previously, coordination among these several bodies is slowly being attempted, but it has not yet been fully achieved in any South American country.

In Chile, where in 1952 a high degree of coordination was attained through the National Health Service, there was also established in 1961 a continental center for studying and training personnel in the field of national health planning. In the Center for Development Studies (CENDES is the Spanish acronym) at Santiago, a special technical approach to planning was formulated by the Pan American Health Organization (PAHO) or regional office of the World Health Organization. The PAHO-CENDES method, as it is called, is based on the establishment of priorities for dealing with specific disease problems on the basis of their death rates, quantified according to their magnitude, importance, and vulnerability.

In the rather complex formulas required to apply this planning method, magnitude is defined by the percentage of all deaths in a nation or a region owing to a specified cause. Importance is determined by the years of potential life lost owing to the death; hence, the death of a young person is deemed more important than the death of an old person. Vulnerability measures the effectiveness with which the disease can be treated or, better yet, prevented. All three factors are quantified and then related to the cost of taking the necessary social action. These calculations are expected to yield both priorities and cost-benefit ratios, and with this information the planner may offer guidance to decision makers in government.

Although some 2,500 persons were trained in the PAHO-CENDES method, it has in fact not been successfully applied anywhere. The statistical information required has generally been unavailable and, moreover, in practice health services are seldom provided on a disease-by-disease or age-specific basis. The value of this training has now come to be regarded mainly as methodological—that is, it indoctrinates health personnel with a sense of quantification, so that future decisions, it is hoped, will be based on some sort of objective rather than purely intuitional or political grounds.

Welfare States

The social insurance systems in the European welfare states have basically involved planning of the economic aspects of access to medical care. As a secondary effect of this sort of planning, the production and use of health manpower and facilities have been indirectly influenced. Pressures for greater economy and higher quality of services, moreover, have led most welfare states to take further actions, of which only a few may be cited.

The organization of the British National Health Service in 1948 and its reorganization in 1974 have been discussed. Implicit in the entire structure, was a planned arrangement for providing the population with (1) primary treatment services of general practitioners, prescribed drugs, dental care, and other ambulatory services, (2) specialist services and care in hospitals, and (3) various preventive and domiciliary services given through resources of local government authorities. The 1974 legislation intended that these several health functions of a publicly supported system should become better coordinated. More deliberate planning of the training of medical specialists, however—to cite just one problem—is being contemplated, so that hospitals will not be confronted with excessive numbers of applicants in some specialties and too few in others. Moreover, the most serious underlying problem in the British health system is probably the small over-all percentage of national wealth being devoted to it—about 5.5 percent of gross national product—in relation to the health needs and demands. It is this basic fact that accounts for the long waiting times for elective hospital admissions or the perfunctory care given by many busy general practitioners. Correction of these problems requires a larger allocation of national resources to the health sector, which involves planning decisions in the whole panorama of social and political priorities.

In Sweden, much of the health planning effort has been devoted to the establishment of efficient networks of hospitals. At the national level, the country has been divided into eight regions, in each of which a full range of treatment services are available. With the familiar pyramidal concept, the most complex services are planned for large and highly specialized regional hospitals, each serving about 1 million people. At the next level are the central county hospitals, serving about 250,000 people for moderately complex conditions. At the most local level are district hospitals of smaller size (about 300 beds) to serve about 75,000 people for the simplest conditions. Each hospital also offers out-patient services, but in addition there would be peripheral health centers for every 10,000 to 20,000 people for ambulatory care. The latter component of the planning is relatively undeveloped, since private medical practice is still strong. Nevertheless, legislation was passed in 1971 that was intended to strengthen the public medical services and weaken the private sector. The exact numbers, location, and specialty distribution of hospital beds of the several types are based on studies of diagnoses in the health insurance records and estimates of the time required for patients to reach a hospital.

Canada has also used its health insurance data to calculate better the proportionate distribution of specialists and family practitioners required to meet population needs. Various expert committees study the health care utilization data and draw conclusions on the numbers of specialists that would be proper in each field, taking account of the optimal time to be spent per case, the expanded use of auxiliary personnel, probable changes in the prevalence of various diseases, and so on. Rising costs in Canada have also led to decisions to reduce the ratio of hospital beds to population, and similarly, the total supply of physicians. There is also deliberate promotion in several provinces of health centers as an approach to greater efficiency in the coordinated delivery of preventive and therapeutic ambulatory services.

Free Enterprise Settings

In the United States, comprehensive health planning became an explicit national strategy with the passing of a federal law in 1966, soon after the enactment of socially insured Medicare for the aged. As in Europe, planning had long been applied to several parts of the health field, such as industrial injury care, services for maternal and child health, hospital construction, and so on, but the 1966 legislation provided grants to local areas for comprehensive health planning.

The hallmark of current American health planning is the vesting of authority principally in numerous separate local bodies. There are no national health care standards that these bodies are obligated to follow, although conditions are set on their administrative structure (e.g., the composition of citizen boards) and their general functions. The original 1966 act has actually expired, along with other closely related legislation on regional medical programs and on hospital construction subsidies, but in 1974 the National Health Planning and Resource Development law was enacted, combining the content of several previous laws.

The National Health Planning and Resource Development law establishes about 200 regions in the United States with populations of 500,000 to 3,000,000. Consistent with the American pluralistic tradition, in each region there will be a Health System Agency (HSA) sponsored by either a local governmental or voluntary body. The planning functions of HSAs may be of very wide scope within their jurisdictions. Such functions include the approval of hospital construction, including supplies and types of beds, the application for and use of federal grants-to-states in several fields (child health, mental health services, venereal disease control, etc.), the training and use of various types of health personnel, the promotion of services for special problems, such as cancer detection, alcoholism, or accident control, arrangement for ambulatory care of the poor, and other tasks. Each state is also to have a State Health Council with general coordinating functions. It is noteworthy, however, that there is no mechanism for the establishment of uniform standards in any field or for national determination of needs. All health planning problems are presumably to be solved independently by 200 autonomous local bodies, with only suggested "guidelines" from higher levels.

In other types of country, where health planning is virtually synonymous with centralized determination of needs and program standards, followed by reasonable allocation of resources, this American approach to planning may seem puzzling. It has greater meaning, however, when considered in conjunction with other legislation being contemplated by the United States federal government. Most important is the legislation for nationwide medical care insurance that is embodied in more than twenty bills introduced in the Congress. When or if one of these bills is enacted, a far stronger system of economic support for personal health services will be in force, and this should enable the local HSAs to carry out their planning functions more effectively. Also under consideration is a new federal program for subsidizing the training of many types of health manpower. Several federal health manpower subsidy laws have been in effect since the 1940s in the United States; without them, the heightened demands for health care associated with the growth of voluntary health insurance could not have been met. The newly contemplated legislation, however, may extend federal support far beyond previous levels. It may also address the crucial problem of allocations among the numerous medical specialties and methods of attaining better geographic distribution of health manpower generally.

Finally, a United States federal law enacted in 1972 has other implications for health planning. This law promoted Health Maintenance Organizations (HMOs). Voluntary health insurance programs, providing a wide range of medical and hospital services for a sum paid periodically in advance (the definition of HMOs), have operated in the United States for years. The new element has been the promotion of such programs by subsidies from the federal government. On the basis of the experience of existing HMOs, there is strong evidence that this mechanism achieves economies in the use of expensive hospitalization, and perhaps in other ways. The reason is evidently that doctors (and others) on HMO staffs have a financial incentive to keep down the rate of hospital days in the enrolled population for which they are responsible. Since the enrollment premium is fixed in advance, less money spent on hospitalization as well as on prescribed drugs or other secondary services leaves more money for payment to the doctors and others. There is, of course, the hazard of underservicing of patients for financial gain, so that some form of governmental surveillance is necessary aside from the protection of competition and patient disenrollment. Assuming the maintenance of quality standards, however, the HMO strategy is an essentially free enterprise approach to health care planning. It provides built-in financial incentives to promote economical use of resources and, under prudent supervision, to encourage the maintenance of health.

Priorities and the Achievement of Equity

Finally, we must consider the determination of priorities in health care systems and the worldwide trends toward achievement of equity. Explicitly or implicitly, every health care system has its priorities, that is, the population groups or health problems that warrant the highest degree of attention. A full exploration of this topic would be an enormous task, but we will take note of some of the highlights.

Insofar as the open market operates, it is evident that in the free enterprise setting the greatest claim on scarce resources goes to those with greatest buying power or personal wealth. In many ways, however, there has been intervention in the free market, and special priorities have been advanced. In the sector of public health services, for example, health promotion for children and expectant mothers have a high priority. So far as voluntary health insurance eases the access to medical care, services in the hospital clearly have the highest priority; this type of insurance benefit protects much greater numbers of people than does insurance for ambulatory care or drugs. With respect to social insurance, the priorities are for the care of occupational injuries (worker's compensation) and the treatment of aged pensioners (Medicare). Among illnesses whose care is financed largely by general revenues, one must recognize the priorities assigned to tuberculosis, serious psychoses, venereal disease, and quite recently grave kidney disease requiring dialysis.

In the welfare states, the highest priorities appear to go to the general medical care of employed workers. Even family dependents, as in Japan, may be less fully protected than the primary worker. In many countries, specialist services in hospitals have been more bountifully financed than primary care services, so that the latter are in declining supply. Still, compared to the United States, the services of general practitioners are more plentiful in the welfare states because of the lesser development of specialization. Access to primary care is becoming recognized as an increasing priority for social insurance protection. Babies and expectant mothers have high priority for public revenue support. Public revenue also supports dental care for children from families of all income.

The transitional countries, with their fractional coverage of the population through social insurance, clearly put high priority on the medical care of regularly employed industrial or mine workers. Dependents are often not protected, and agricultural workers, generally in surplus supply, get much smaller per capita outlays for health care. The small top social class enjoys relatively luxurious medical services from personal physicians and in private hospitals. In the rural areas, major attention goes to the reduction of infant mortality and to campaigns against specific diseases such as malaria, yellow fever, and tuberculosis.

National campaigns against communicable diseases have a high priority in the severely underdeveloped countries. Programs against tropical vector-borne diseases are an object of major international assistance, as are various strategies to promote birth control. As in the transitional countries, an elite class in the main cities gets highly favored attention, along with the military forces and higher government officials. For political reasons and also to create an impressive national image, excessive expenditures are made on a few monumental hospitals in the capital cities. On the other hand, increasing efforts have recently been put into the training of auxiliary health aides for the rural villages.

In the socialist countries influenced by the Soviet Union, the highest priority is clearly assigned to industrial workers. The central thrust of the over-all planning strategy has been industrialization. Protection and promotion of the health of children are also major emphases, expressed in the education of medical personnel and the construction of facilities, as well as in the provision of treatment and preventive services. Among the sectors of medical care, drugs in the socialist systems get less support than in the welfare states; they must still be largely purchased privately, in spite of the public support of physician and hospital services. In the People's Republic of China, since 1965, the major priority has clearly been assigned to the vast rural population; the massive training of barefoot doctors and the establishment of thousands of health stations in the rural communes have been the prominent strategy.

Identification of priorities for health service in a country is not easy, for judgments must be made along several dimensions: (1) sectors of the population according to social class, place of residence (urban or rural), age level, and other attributes; (2) types of disease, such as communicable, metabolic, nutritional, traumatic, or other features; (3) forms of service, as among hospital-based, ambulatory care, prevention, pharmaceutical, and so on. There are, furthermore, combinations of priority choices along two or three of these dimensions of health need that may attract proportionately high allocations of resources, such as preventive services for children in rural areas or treatment in hospitals of aged persons in large cities. The determinants of priorities, in the face of invariably deficient resources, are complex combinations of political and economic forces. As noted, moreover, some priority decisions are made deliberately by public authorities in the context of national health planning; other priorities occur, in a sense, by default, insofar as free market dynamics are not touched and health services follow the flow of dollars from different individuals.

In spite of these variations in the allocation of resources for health care, one can detect in all five types of country the acceleration of social pressures for achieving greater equity in the distribution of health services. Matters affecting life and death obviously have strong political significance, and governments that may hesitate to launch changes in other spheres will often take action to improve the general availability of health care.

Thus, in virtually all countries, we see a movement to increase the total resources—manpower, facilities, and equipment—for health services, and an increasing share of the cost of financing those resources is being derived through collective channels such as government or charity or various sorts of insurance. This very process renders health care spending more visible and leads invariably to greater concern for efficiency; the money should be wisely spent. In practical terms, this usually means an increasingly rationalized use of manpower in health teams, where the division of labor can improve the cost-benefit ratio. The services also must be made accessible geographically as well as economically. And finally, as populations become more sophisticated about the health sciences, they demand greater surveillance over the quality of their application. Regulatory controls on the performance of health care providers are increased.

All these movements lead to the more equitable distribution of health services, that is, their provision in relation to individual needs as distinguished from private purchasing power. The pace of these movements differs among the several types of country. It certainly does not proceed smoothly; political events can lead to sudden spurts in the process of achieving health equity. There may even be some movement backward at times, although the long-term trend is clearly toward an egalitarian ideal. Health service, like the availability of food, is a fundamental need for survival that no type of political leadership can ignore. Regardless of the dominant ideology, from the most individualistic to the most socialistic, ways are being found to increase the population's accessibility to health care. The free economic market is modified or interceded in for health objectives more readily than for many other services or commodities. Despite the social conflicts that this often generates, it seems that the political payoffs almost everywhere are considered worth the problems.

At this moment, of course, the progress that has been made toward a truly egalitarian concept of equity varies greatly among countries. If we randomly chose 1,000 Americans and could quantify their receipt of health services—as among the wealthy, the moderately affluent, the marginally poor, and the very poor—we would find great differentials that would be much greater than a similar examination of 1,000 persons from Sweden, Great Britain, or the USSR. On the other hand, the equity among the 1,000 Americans would be far greater today than it was in 1930 or in 1900. Likewise, in the three other countries mentioned, the distribution of health services would still be far from perfectly equitable. Even under the British National Health Service, the wealthy, for reasons of knowledge, sophistication, access to transportation, the attitudes of providers, and other factors, obtain more of the health services they need than do the poor. The point is, however, that in *all* types of country, although in varying degrees, the distribution of services on the basis of need rather than personal affluence is becoming more equalized.

As we look around the world, furthermore, we see increasingly similar patterns in the organization and delivery of health services. Although this book has, in a sense, underscored the differences among various types of country, the global view also shows great commonalities. The private group practice clinic in the United States and the public polyclinic in the Soviet Union have similarities as well as differences. The United States' voluntary Blue Cross plans have traits matched in the governmental health service of New Zealand, as well as contrasts. Through it all, the demands of people and the technology of health science are apparently driving the social forms of health service organization in a common direction. Each country, as suggested at the outset, may be regarded as a laboratory where different sets of factors are at play and their effects are being tested. To say that each country can learn something from every other country is not a cliché. The overriding conclusion is that there is a ferment in all health care systems toward the achievement of increasing equity in the access of people to the human benefits of science.

Readings

Abel-Smith, Brian, "Health Priorities in Developing Countries: The Economist's Contribution," *International Journal of Health Services,* 2:5-12 (1972).

Anderson, Odin W., *Health Care: Can There Be Equity—United States, Sweden, and England,* New York: John Wiley & Sons, 1972.

Battistella, Roger M. and T. E. Chester, "Role of Management in Health Services in Britain and the United States," *The Lancet,* 18 March 1972, pp. 626-629.

Desta, A., "An Approach to National Health Planning," *Ethiopian Medical Journal, 10*:71-74 (April 1972).

Elling, Ray H., "Health Planning in International Perspective," *Medical Care, 9*:214-234 (May-June 1971).

Elling, Ray (ed.), *Health Systems and Health Planning in International Perspective—An Annotated Bibliography*, Monticello, Ill.: Council of Planning Librarians, Exchange Bibliography No. 265, March 1972.

Engel, Arthur, *Perspectives in Health Planning*, London: Athlone Press, 1968.

Fendall, N. R. E., "Planning Health Services in Developing Countries," *Public Health Reports, 78*:977-988 (November 1963).

Haraldson, S., "Appraisal of Health Problems and Definition of Priorities in Health Planning," *Ethiopian Medical Journal, 37*:37-44 (1970).

Haro, A. S. and T. Purola, "Planning and Health Policy in Finland," *International Journal of Health Services, 2*:23-34 (1972).

Harding, C. D., "Area-wide Health Planning in Latin America," *World Hospitals, 6*:5-11 (1970).

Hilleboe, H. E., A. Barkhuus, and W. C. Thomas, Jr., *Approaches to National Health Planning*, Geneva: World Health Organization, Public Health Papers No. 46, 1972.

Litsios, S., "The Principles and Methods of Evaluation of National Health Plans," *International Journal of Health Services, 1*:79-85 (1971).

Logan, Robert F. L., "National Health Planning: An Appraisal of the State of the Art," *International Journal of Health Services, 1*:6-17 (February 1971).

MacLeod, Gordon, "A Critical Commentary on Consumerism in Denamrk and the United States," *Scandinavian Review*, September 1975.

Martin, Jean F., "International Health Planning: Socioenvironmental Dimensions and Community Participation," *Americal Journal of Public Health, 65*:175-177 (February 1975).

Mercenier, P., "Methodology of Health Planning in Developing Countries," *Transactions of the Royal Society of Tropical Medicine and Hygiene, 65*:40-46 (supplement) (1971).

Morley, David C., *Pediatric Priorities in the Developing World*, Toronto: Butterworths, 1973.

Navarro, Vicente, "Health, Health Services, and Health Planning in Cuba," *International Journal of Health Services, 2*:397-432 (1972).

———, *National and Regional Health Planning in Sweden*, Washington, D.C.: U.S. Department of Health, Education, and Welfare, 1974.

Pan American Health Organization, *Health Planning in Latin America*, Washington, D.C.: PAHO Scientific Pub. No. 272, 1973.

Pizam, A. and I. Meir, "The Management of Health Care Organizations—Medical vs. Administrative Orientation: The Case of Kupat Holim," *Medical Care, 12*:682-692 (August 1974).

Poldermans, J. D. G., "Statistics and Planning in the Health Services of West Germany and the United Kingdom," *Social Science and Medicine, 5*:339-361 (August 1971).

Popov, G. A., *Principles of Health Planning in the USSR*, Geneva: World Health Organization, Public Health Papers No. 43, 1971.

Roemer, Milton I., "Medical Care and Social Class in Latin America," *Milbank Memorial Fund Quarterly, 42*:54-64 (1964).

——, "Planning Health Services: Substance versus Form," *Canadian Journal of Public Health, 59*:431-437 (November 1968).

Sanazaro, Paul J., "International Health Services Research" in Evelyn Flook and Paul J. Sanazaro (eds.), *Health Services Research and R & D in Perspective,* Ann Arbor, Mich.: Health Administration Press, 1973.

Scrimshaw, Nevin S., "Myths and Realities in International Health Planning," *American Journal of Public Health, 64*:792-798 (August 1974).

Skrbkova, Emilie and Milos Vacek, "Some Problems in Health Care Organization in Czechoslovakia," *Medical Care, 9*:405-414 (September-October 1971).

Somers, Anne R., "The Rationalization of Health Services: A Universal Priority," *Inquiry, 8*:48-60 (March 1971).

Webster, M. G., "Health Service Administration in Developing Countries," *South African Medical Journal, 43*:1043-1046 (1969).

Weinerman, E. Richard, *Social Medicine in Eastern Europe,* Cambridge, Mass.: Harvard University Press, 1969.

World Bank, *Health* (Sector Policy Paper), Washington, D.C.: World Bank, March 1975.

World Health Organization, *National Health Planning in Developing Countries,* Geneva: WHO Tech. Report Series No. 350, 1967.

World Health Organization, Regional Office for Europe, *Planning and Evaluating Dental Health Services,* Copenhagen: WHO, 1972.

World Health Organization, *Modern Management Methods and the Organization of Health Services,* Geneva: WHO, 1974.

World Health Organization, *Fifth Report of the World Health Situation 1969-1972, Geneva: WHO, 1975.*

10

SOME NATIONAL HEALTH SYSTEM PANORAMAS

Having reviewed the main features of health care systems in different types of country of the world, it may now be helpful to see how these features tie together in a country. The exact linkages among the features and the resultant configurations differ, of course, in all nations because of the diverse historical backgrounds, economic levels, political policies, and other cultural factors at play. Obviously, no two countries are exactly alike in their health care systems or anything else.

We have tried to simplify an analysis of some 150 nations, however, by clustering them into five types classified along broad economic and political lines. Despite variations even within types, we will select one country of each type and summarize briefly the panoramas of five contrasting health care systems.

A Free Enterprise System—The United States

In spite of the rapid changes occurring in the health care system of the United States, it most nearly epitomizes the free enterprise concept of a health care system relative to other countries of the world. More prominently than elsewhere, the provision of health services is influenced by an open economic market, even though one may observe daily increasing interventions in that market by governmental and also private actions that are designed to achieve greater equity in the distribution of health services.

As the world's most affluent nation, the United States allocates a rising proportion of an enlarging gross national product (GNP) for health purposes. In 1975 over 8 percent of the United States' GNP was being spent for health, including construction of health facilities and medical research, as well as health services. This expenditure did not include education of health personnel, considered part of education costs. The greatest share, about 40 percent, pays for hospital care, approximately 25 percent for physician services, and the balance for dental care, drugs, and so on as well as for organized preventive services, research, and other purposes. With respect to sources of support, about 40 percent now comes from government agencies, including social insurance programs at federal (Medicare) and state (industrial injury compensation) levels. Approximately another 20 percent is channeled through voluntary health insurance programs, about 35 percent through purely private payments, and the balance (5 percent) through charity and industry.

Most of the collectivized mechanisms of financing support hospital services, general care of the poor, the military and other selected populations, the treatment of mental illness, organized prevention, facility construction, and medical research. Voluntary insurance is also largely directed toward hospital services and physician services in the hospital. Private payment is the chief source of support of ambulatory medical services, dental care, drugs (prescribed and nonprescribed), eyeglasses, and other aspects of health care. The trend, however, has been prominently toward increased collectivization of economic support in all sectors and with this a rising degree of social discipline in the operations of the entire health care system.

To provide these services, a mounting proportion of the American labor force is devoted to the health field. In 1975, counting all types of personnel in the health industry, about 5 million persons were so involved, or about one out of every sixteen persons in the nation's actively employed population of some 80 million. Of these 5 million about 330,000 are doctors; the great majority are nurses, pharmacists, technicians, and many other types of allied health personnel. Among the doctors, about 80 percent are specialists, resulting in only about 20 percent general practitioners, a keenly felt shortage. Deficiencies of health manpower are found particularly in low-income sections of the large cities and in rural areas. To cope with these problems, increasing interest has developed in recent years in training physician assistants, nurse practitioners, and other forms of replacement for the doctor—mainly for primary health care.

General hospitals are predominantly under the control of local, autonomous voluntary bodies. Government sponsorship of general hospitals (about 33 percent of the beds) is mainly at the municipal or county level, although mental hospitals are sponsored mainly by state governments. Somewhat over half of the eight total hospital beds per 1,000 population are in general facilities, and the balance are in special institutions for the mentally ill or for persons with other long-term disease. In addition, there is a large supply of nursing homes for the primarily custodial care (but with some skilled nursing) of the aged who have chronic disabilities. Health centers for organized ambulatory care are relatively few, and usually function as places to house public health (typically prevention-oriented) agencies or to serve selected low-income populations. Pharmacies are virtually all private businesses, as are the premises of practicing physicians, dentists, and most other health care providers.

The pattern of delivery of general medical care—services for diagnosis and treatment of most disease—is predominantly private. Most doctors and nearly all dentists work in their own private offices. Even when economic support has been assumed by government or spread through health insurance, the service is usually delivered in private and individual settings. Nevertheless, there has been an accelerating growth of group practice among private doctors, and a rising share of ambulatory services is being furnished at hospital outpatient departments and certain other organized settings. Specialty services are delivered both in private offices and hospitals, but only a small proportion of specialists—mainly pathologists, radiologists, and anesthesiologists—are on full-time salaries in general hospitals. (This does not count many thousands of young doctors in training programs in hospitals.) For their work both outside and inside hospitals, the great majority of doctors are paid on a fee-for-service basis, even though the fraction paid by salaries has been increasing. Medical incomes are extremely high relative to those of other occupational groups, and the earnings of other types of health personnel have also been rising.

Preventive health services in the United States are highly developed with respect to environmental protection. Water supply and excreta disposal are almost entirely through public systems, and diseases spread by water or food, as well as by insect vectors, have been reduced to low levels. Preventive services to children and expectant mothers are given mainly through private arrangements, even though there are also numerous clinics for such services that are used especially by the poor. Family planning services are likewise mainly furnished by private doctors, although public clinics for this purpose have been rapidly increasing. Because of the mounting importance of the chronic diseases of later life in causing both disability and mortality, increasing efforts have been put into early detection of these disorders and into epidemiological research that might point to measures of primary prevention.

The most pervasive form of regulation of the health care system is through licensure of health personnel by state governments, but many other approaches are growing. Hospitals are licensed by the states and are also accredited by a national voluntary body. The medical and surgical specialties are certified by private professional bodies to provide standards for training and tests for competence. Hospitals have developed increasing forms of discipline over the performance of their medical staffs. Programs of governmentally financed health service have required a widening range of peer review procedures to monitor quality and costs. The pharmaceutical industry, which is entirely private, has been subjected to expanding controls over the production, marketing (including advertising), and distribution of their products, largely in response to tragedies caused by toxic drugs. Patients are exercising increasing influence on the performance of health care providers through court actions for malpractice and through a movement for consumer participation in policy decisions on health programs.

The over-all administrative structure of the health care system in the United States is often called pluralistic. Authority is very much decentralized within government, and nongovernmental or voluntary bodies also exercise great power and influence. There are enormous diversities in the patterns of both the financing and delivery of health services in different states or even different sections of one state. Systematic planning of health resources and services has been increasing, but it also is still principally on a decentralized basis. Even though the role of the national government in both health service programs and in health planning has been steadily mounting, it is mediated largely through federal grants to the states or even to local voluntary bodies. Social and political forces are driving the American health care system toward greater coordination and central controls, but for the present, relative to other nations, the priorities in health care delivery are determined mainly by personal wealth.

A Welfare State System—Norway

In the welfare state category of country, there are many variations, but all such countries are characterized by having the great bulk of their health services financed through collective channels. With this are associated many features of health care delivery that contrast with conditions in the United States. A panorama of this type of system is illustrated by Norway.

Data on the precise distribution of expenditures for health purposes are not so readily available for Norway as for the United States, but the total proportion of GNP devoted to health is somewhat less, about 6 to 7 percent. Of this amount, 50 percent goes to the support of hospital services, even more than in the United States. To some extent, though, this is misleading, since Norwegian cost data count the services of in-hospital doctors as part of hospital costs, whereas American national accounting does not. Still the rate of general hospital days per 1,000 population in Norway is somewhat higher (about 1,400 days per 1,000 in Norwegian general hospitals compared with 1,200 days per 1,000 in American), and the relative expenditures on other services, such as drugs and research, are lower.

More reflective of the general character of the Norwegian system is the high percentage of economic support for health services coming from collective sources. Social insurance for almost complete medical care covers 100 percent of the population. Hospital services are financed 75 percent by the social insurance system and 25 percent by local county governments; the patient pays nothing, except for special amenities, such as a private room, for which the extra charges are low. Outside the hospital, physician's care and drugs require 20 percent co-payments by the patient (or cost sharing) on the first three visits but not on continuing treatment of chronic illness, nor are there any charges for pensioners or the very poor. Publicly financed dental services are highly developed for school children of all income levels, although adults must pay privately. Altogether one may estimate that about 80 percent of health care costs in Norway are borne by social insurance and government revenues (roughly 50 percent from the former and 30 percent from the latter). Of the remaining 20 percent, some comes from charity and industry, a trifle from voluntary insurance, and about 15 percent of the total from private payments.

The Norwegian supply of doctors is about the same as that in the United States, with a ratio of about 1:650. The distribution between general practitioners and specialists, however, differs significantly—about 40 percent being in general practice and 60 percent in the specialties. The supply of nurses at all levels is about the same as in the United States, at about 1:185. However, nurses are often called on to perform a wider range of functions in hospitals, such as laboratory and x-ray technology, medical record work, and other activities done typically by special allied personnel in the United States. More important perhaps is the major reliance in Norway on nurses specifically trained for the tasks to perform midwifery and anesthesia functions. Virtually all normal maternity cases are delivered in hospitals by nurse-midwives, and all except the most complex surgical anesthesia cases are handled by nurse-anesthetists under a medical anesthesiologist's general supervision.

On the other hand, nurses are not being trained as nurse-practitioners in the American sense, nor are there any physician assistants. Primary care is regarded as the unique responsibility of a general medical practitioner, who may be aided by a nurse for certain procedures (such as blood pressure determinations or injections) but who is never replaced as a decision maker. The Norwegian GP, one must realize, is not only in relatively greater supply than the American, but he is regarded as having a much more important role in general patient care. He has few if any ties to hospitals but gets his prestige and rewards from his ties to families. If a patient requires specialist care or hospitalization, he is sent to a hospital doctor, and then returns to his general practitioner after discharge, with a summary of the in-hospital experience being sent to the GP.

Dentists are in greater relative supply in Norway than in the United States —about 1 to 1200 population, compared to 1 to 2000 in America. (This is unusual, however, among the welfare states, most of whom have a smaller supply of dentists than the United States.) Accordingly, there is no problem in filling the salaried posts in the highly developed public dental services for school children and certain other age groups that are financed by both local and national governments. With the abundance of dentists, there has also been no pressure to develop middle-level dental personnel, such as the New Zealand-style dental nurse, for giving both therapeutic and preventive dental service to children.

Hospitals in Norway are overwhelmingly owned and operated by units of government, mostly local. About 90 percent of general hospital beds and even higher proportions of mental or other special beds are in government facilities. As in most of western Europe, the staffing is more modest than in the United States, with about 1.5 personnel per bed in a hospital of the size (around 200 beds) that in the United States would have 2.5 personnel per bed. The hospital board is typically appointed by elected officials or sometimes directly elected. Top executive responsibility is usually carried by a salaried physician, who is assisted by a business manager. The nonmedical hospital administrator prevalent in the United States is rarely found at the top of the organizational structure.

Most markedly different from American patterns is the mode of work of doctors in hospitals. Practically all in-hospital service is provided by salaried specialists, usually full-time, although a small share of the time of some may be spent outside in private offices. Specialist salaries are relatively high, and the posts carry great prestige. When an opening occurs, it is advertised and is subject to competition. Nominations are made by the Director-General of Health Services in the national Ministry of Social Affairs, and one of these is appointed by the local County Council. All hospitals have well-developed outpatient departments where the specialists examine and treat patients referred typically by a general practitioner.

One can appreciate how this system leads to a lower proportion of specialists than the open-market American setting. The number of Norwegian specialists in orthopedic surgery, for example, will depend largely on the number of hospital beds set up for this type of case. To be admitted to a hospital bed, the patient must not only be referred by his family doctor but also must be reviewed by a hospital doctor who, being on salary, has no financial incentive to admit the case. Medical need is the only criterion. Accordingly, the rate of hospital admissions is lower than in the United States, but the average lengths of stay are longer, so that aggregate hospital days per 1,000 are greater. Under these circumstances, Norway finds that having 60 percent of its doctors in specialty practice is quite enough.

Outside the hospital, specialization is rare except for the part-time activities of doctors based in a hospital. However, as noted, general practice is much more highly developed. Although more than 80 percent of GP income is derived from payments from the social insurance system (made through a local insurance office), the remuneration is on a fee-for-service basis. An official fee schedule is followed, with cost sharing by the patient, as explained earlier. The majority of community doctors practice alone, but in recent years partnerships of two, three, or four—all general practitioners—have been forming more frequently. In some communities, local governments have built health centers where GPs rent space, work together in a small team, and have the assistance of nurses, social workers, technicians, or other allied personnel.

To assure primary health care for Norway's large rural stretches with thinly settled populations there is a network of official district doctors with a wide range of duties. These positions are under the national Directorate of Health Services, with a basic salary being paid for various preventive services—communicable disease control, school and maternal-infant health services, forensic medicine, supervision of environmental sanitation, and so on. Most of the district doctor's income, however, comes from social insurance fees paid for general medical care rendered to the people in his district. Being in an official post, the doctor (usually young) entering one of these positions becomes immediately known to the local population. Moreover, since he has been appointed by a national authority, his qualifications are respected. For some years, all new qualified Norwegian medical graduates were obligated to serve in a district doctor post for two years, but since 1970 the medical school output has been so increased and the positions have become so attractive that all such jobs have been filled voluntarily.

Preventive health services in the cities of Norway are similar in type to those in the United States, but they are different in extent. Most striking is the great development of public health clinics for child health promotion. Instead of serving mainly the children of poor families, these clinics serve about 90 percent of all infants in their first year of life; specially trained nurses do most of the work, with a doctor in periodic attendance. Clinics for tuberculosis and venereal disease control are also well developed. As noted earlier, dental services—both preventive and restorative—for school children are provided at government expense throughout the nation.

Regulation of the quality of health services in Norway rests more on government control of the medical schools and other training institutions than on subsequent licensure hurdles. In fact, after graduation from an approved school, registration of the health professional with the Ministry of Social Affairs is merely a formality. The schools, moreover, are financed almost entirely by government funds, so that student tuition payments are insignificant. Specialty qualifications in medicine, however, are supervised by the nongovernment Norwegian Medical Association, which establishes requirements for postgraduate training and certifies doctors in the several specialty fields.

The peer review approach to monitoring medical performance, based largely on examining medical records, that is so current in the United States is not seen in Norway. The health insurance bodies monitor fee claims that suggest deviant medical practice—such as exceptionally high rates of prescriptions or excessive consultations per case—and may call on the doctor involved for an explanation. In hospitals, however, where the most complex medical work is done, the whole framework of service is organized. Group discipline, in a sense, is part of daily activity and need not be exercised ex post facto, as in the American hospital. Even the district doctors doing community general practice are subject to surveillance by the national Directorate of Health Services.

Likewise, the control of drugs is not so dependent as in the United States on surveillance over manufacturing and marketing. Most drugs are imported, and the Directorate of Health Services controls the number and types of drugs that may enter or be sold in the country; the current approved list numbers only about 2,000, compared with tens of thousands in the United States. Moreover, pharmacies come under government supervision. Although they are privately owned, they must meet certain standards, and a new pharmacy may be established only with official approval. If an area is deemed well supplied with pharmacies, new ones are prohibited, and the prospective pharmaceutical merchant must open his business somewhere else in need of drug service or become employed by an existing pharmacy.

Administratively it is quite apparent that the authority of government in general, and especially national government, is much greater in the Norwegian welfare state setting than in the United States. Voluntary health agencies play a part, but they are mainly to provide volunteer services rather than to raise money. In fact, most voluntary agencies—for example, those concerned with the care of retarded children— are subsidized by government grants. Local government plays a significant role in operating hospitals, but national standards must be met. Consumerism is not a prominent movement, as we see it currently in the United States, because elected officials already control hospitals, workers or other consumer groups control the social insurance organizations, and the whole parliamentary structure of government depends, of course, on the voting process. Thus, the Minister of Social Affairs, under whom comes the Directorate of Health Services, must be a member of Parliament elected from some district. Patient satisfaction with the whole system is very high. Litigation for malpractice is rare.

Health planning is part of the normal operations of the health insurance system, of the educational institutions turning out health manpower (under the Ministry of Church and Education), and of the whole wide range of preventive and other services under the Directorate of Health Services. In recent years, the functions of hospitals have been more deliberately planned according to the concept of regionalization—that is, with responsibilities for cases scaled among facilities of small, intermediate, and large size. With hospital costs rising rapidly in Norway as everywhere, more emphasis is being directed to ambulatory care through greater strengthening of general practice. Continuing education of general practitioners is stressed, as well as providing GPs with auxiliary personnel and building health centers in which they can work more effectively.

It is hard to identify priorities in Norwegian health services, since practically all types of care are financially supported for everyone. Insofar as public revenue support implies a greater social commitment than health insurance mechanisms, one may say that small children are a high priority for total health care, including dental service. Primary care of the rural population gets major and deliberate attention through the district doctor system. At the same time, hospitals are well supported by both social insurance and general revenue sources. In terms of the most recent emphasis, however, the priority pendulum seems to be swinging toward integrated preventive and curative primary care with the promotion of health service teams in health centers.

A Transitional System—Peru

As applies to most transitional countries of Latin America, health services in Peru reflect several historical influences. The original Indian culture gave rise to traditional healing practices that are still found widely in the rural areas. The Catholic church of Spain gave rise to many charitable or *beneficencia* hospitals for the care of the urban poor. North American influence promoted public health programs, especially through environmental sanitation and mass campaigns against certain vector-borne diseases. Finally, modern Europe disseminated the social security idea and gave rise to a special subsystem of health services for insured workers. At the same time, as a class of wealthy or even middle-class families developed, mainly in the large cities, a private medical care sector took root.

Thus today the economic support for health services in Peru is quite diversified. The total percentage of the GNP devoted to health purposes is not known, but since Peru is a generally agricultural and developing economy with much lower per capita income than any of the European countries, this percentage is probably low, perhaps around 3 percent. For the great majority of the population, considering the services of scientific medicine, health care is financed predominantly from collective sources, that is, from general revenues mainly at the national level, from social security contributions, and from charitable donations. However, from the viewpoint of the money actually spent, a great deal (one can estimate from studies in other Latin American countries that it is about 50 per cent) comes from private payments that are of two sorts. There are those made by poor villagers for the services of traditional healers or *curanderos*. And there are relatively large sums paid by a very small fraction of the people who are affluent—perhaps 5 to 10 percent of the population—for the services of private doctors or for private rooms in hospitals. With the latter, one must count also the cost of privately purchased drugs and dental care. Thus, the expenditure of money has uneven and inequitable impacts on the population. Although these figures are only approximations, the basic idea is that—leaving aside traditional nonscientific healing—about 50 percent of the health money goes for the care of about 10 percent of the population, while the other 50 percent must serve the needs of 90 percent of the population.

Moreover, within the collectivized 50 percent of expenditures, there are further imbalances in the amplitude with which they affect the 90 percent of Peruvians who are of low income. A fortunate 27 percent of the work force, but only about 15 percent of the total population, are regularly employed and covered for medical care by the social security system. This 15 percent of the people receive health benefits financed by social insurance funds, which constitute about half of the collectivized 50 percent of expenditures, or 25 percent of the total. The other half of collectively derived funds (also 25 percent of the total) are used for support of the Ministry of Health program, the charitable (*beneficencia*) hospitals, and some limited municipal services. These latter programs must cope with the needs of the noninsured and nonaffluent masses of the people who constitute about 75 percent of the total Peruvian population. Thus, in an aggregated sense, about 25 percent of all Peruvian expenditures for health services are devoted to organized programs intended to serve 75 percent of the population, whereas 75 percent of the health monies (private payments and social insurance) are concentrated on services to the affluent and the social security beneficiaries.

Even within the social security sector (reaching 15 percent of the population) there are further imbalances since in Peru, as in several Latin American countries, there have been multiple subsystems of social security for manual workers as distinguished from white-collar employees. The latter, with higher salaries, build up larger insurance funds that have been used to support better quality, even elegant, hospital services than can be financed by the insurance derived from manual workers' wages. To satisfy the demands of the doctors as well as the upwardly mobile white-collar employees, moreover, physicians' care may be obtained in private offices rather than polyclinics if the patient is willing to co-pay a share of the medical fee. Quite recently, under Peru's somewhat leftward leaning government, these special disparities within the social security framework have been reduced but not completely eliminated.

Although the above figures on financing health services in Peru are necessarily estimates, they are probably a fair characterization of the uneven distribution of economic support for health care in this transitional Latin American country. With these disparities, there naturally follow great inequities in the quantity and quality of health services provided to different population groups.

Health manpower in Peru corresponds in its availability to the inequities in distribution of health expenditures—that is, more and better trained personnel serve the high income minority and vice versa. Yet, as in transitional countries generally, the manpower supply has been increasing quite rapidly. The ratio of physicians to population, for example improved from 1:4,500 in 1952 to 1: 1,920 in 1969. The supply of dentists, however, is still very poor at 1:6,080, and the supply of pharmacists is 1:6,090. Typical of the situation in most developing countries is the ratio of nurses, being poorer in Peru than that of physicians. at 1:3,200 in 1969. (It will be recalled that in both free enterprise and welfare state countries, there are relatively more nurses than doctors.) Moreover, these data on nurses from the World Health Organization combine both fully trained graduate nurses (equivalent to the RN in Europe or America) and middle-level nursing assistants.

The numbers of traditional healers in Peru are not known, but we can be sure that in the Indian villages of the Andes mountains they are far more numerous than doctors or other scientifically trained personnel. In lesser proportions, the *curanderos* are also found elsewhere in the nation, including even the main cities. Among the nursing personnel, moreover, the more fully trained are largely concentrated in urban hospitals, serving as providers of nursing care to bedpatients and as assistants to doctors. The lesser trained nursing auxiliaries, paradoxically, are more numerous in the rural villages, staffing health stations and health centers; there, with only minimal medical supervision, they usually perform a wider range of duties, including the diagnosis and treatment of common ailments.

Specialization in medicine is much less common in Peru than in the industrialized countries, characterizing perhaps about 25 percent of the doctors. These specialists are almost entirely confined to the main cities, particularly to the national capital, Lima. They all have hospital appointments, often in two or more institutions. Here they serve the poor for part-time salaries and the affluent for private fees. A share of their time, however, is usually spent in private office practice serving the well-to-do.

The geographic distribution of *all* doctors in Peru—general practitioners as well as specialists—is extremely uneven. The Lima metropolitan area contains about 20 percent of the national population but has about 65 percent of all the physicians. Even greater imbalances characterize the distribution of dentists. Pharmacists are also concentrated in the main cities, and in the villages drugs are dispensed at many stores where no pharmacist is on hand.

In contrast to Asian and African countries, where colonial medical systems were only recently displaced, Peru has not made much use of deliberately trained middle-level health personnel to serve as doctor substitutes. With the increasing consciousness, however, of the unmet needs of rural populations, dramatized by the rise of revolutionary guerilla movements, this attitude has been changing. Especially since the Cuban Revolution of 1959, systematic training programs for rural medical assistants have been started in Peru, as in Venezuela (with its *medicina simplificada*), Ecuador, Panama, and some other Latin American countries. Sometimes these medical assistants are men (occasionally former traditional healers), as in Africa or southeast Asia, but more often they are young women. New Peruvian medical graduates are also required to spend a year at a health center or hospital in a rural region.

The hospitals of Peru vary in their design and amenities with the sources of economic support summarized earlier. The total supply of beds is much lower than in the industrialized countries, at about 1.5 beds per 1,000, counting general and special facilities and all types of sponsorship. The majority of the population are served in large, open wards of rather old and meagerly staffed and equipped charitable *beneficencia* hospitals. These are, however, increasingly being re-placed by more modern hospitals of the Ministry of Health, although beds in large multibed wards still outnumber those in semiprivate or private rooms. For social security beneficiaries, the hospitals are of much higher standards. Not only are the beds in smaller wards, with greater space per bed, but facilities for laboratory and x-ray work, for surgery, pharmacy, outpatient service, and so on are much more spacious and better designed. The ratio of beds per 1,000 insured persons, furthermore, is much higher than that for the general population. Mili-tary personnel and sometimes the employees of large industrial establishments are also served by special hospitals, which are generally very well staffed and equipped.

Small private hospitals or *clinicas privadas* are available for serving the affluent minority of the Peruvian population in the main cities. These clinics are typically owned by doctors but sometimes by private societies of prosperous families. In addition, most of the government and *beneficencia* hospitals also maintain a small number of well-furnished rooms for private patients (although this is not done by the social security hospitals). It is not uncommon to observe low-income patients crowded in beds along the corridors of these public hospi-tals, while half the private one- or two-bed rooms are empty.

The financing of hospitals in Peru corresponds largely to their ownership, with one important exception. The charitable hospitals, although owned by church-related welfare societies, are supported mainly by grants from the central government. With these grants has gone an increasing degree of supervision. Thus, the *beneficencia* and the Ministry of Health hospitals are regarded as a net-work that is increasingly being planned and operated along regionalized lines. Likewise, the social security hospitals follow their own regionalization schemes. The newer hospitals of all sponsorships tend to be better designed and equipped for outpatient services. In the rural regions, ambulatory care health centers often serve as satellites to hospitals.

The subsystems for delivery of medical care in Peru are perhaps self-evident from what has already been said. It should only be emphasized that, outside the purely private sector, ambulatory care is given mainly in health centers by salaried doctors and allied personnel, which applies to the socially insured population as well as to the majority who are not so protected. In the rural regions or small towns, health centers are staffed by general medical practitioners and auxiliary personnel. In the larger cities, they have several types of specialist as well, par-ticularly the health centers of the social security agency.

Because of the general poverty of the population, only 15 to 20 percent of the doctors in Peru can earn a living solely from private practice. At least 80 percent have employment, on part-time or full-time salaries, in one or another of the organized health care programs. Insofar as specialty services are obtained by the vast majority of the population, including the socially insured, it is at the outpatient departments of hospitals or polyclinics.

Preventive environmental protection in Peru is poorly developed outside the main cities. For water supply and excreta disposal, most of the population, being rural, are not served by public systems. The Ministry of Health has promoted construction of sanitary wells and latrines, but even such facilities have not yet reached most rural people. Because of the high altitude and relatively cool climate of most of Peru, insect-borne diseases are not a serious problem for environmental control.

As for personal preventive services in Peru, they are well integrated with treatment services in the health centers of all types of sponsorship. Except for the very wealthy, immunizations or preventive maternal and child health services are sought in these public facilities. Tuberculosis is still a significant problem, being dealt with through mass x-ray detection and BCG vaccination of infants under the auspices of the Ministry of Health. Family planning is not officially promoted in Peru, largely because of religious objections, although it is available from private doctors for those who can afford it. Yet many patients on the maternity wards of public hospitals are cases of complications resulting from illegal and improperly performed abortions.

The regulation of health personnel through registration is a function of the Peruvian Ministry of Health, and it depends ordinarily on graduation from an approved university or school, nearly all of which are financed by the central government. Very few foreign professional graduates enter Peru, but those who do may be authorized to practice on the basis of review of their training credentials by the Ministry of Health, which also supervises the production and distribution of drugs. The great majority of drugs are imported, and little is done to ascertain their quality, in spite of the recent disclosure that many outdated medications are "dumped" by American pharmaceutical companies on the Latin American market. The control of drug distribution is especially lax, and patients may purchase almost any type of drug in a pharmacy, with or without a medical prescription.

Hospital regulation by the Ministry of Health is essentially confined to the facilities of the ministry itself and the *beneficencia* societies. Little is done to supervise standards in the social security or private hospitals, although the standards of structure and operation of these are probably in lesser need of surveillance.

Finally, as for the general administrative structure of health services in Peru, it is relatively centralized. Local government is weak, and public authority is exercised principally from Lima. The country is divided into twenty health areas covering twenty four provinces, and the director of each is appointed by the central Ministry of Health. Yet, this area official has no responsibility for social security health activities in his region. Such activities are controlled by a separate central authority.

Health service planning is also a function of the Ministry of Health. Planning has been somewhat effective in getting a network of rural health centers established. Evidently this has been at the expense of hospital construction, since the ratio of hospital beds to population in Peru actually declined between 1960 and 1970. Aside from the mandatory rural service for new medical graduates, however, Peruvian health planning has not significantly intervened in the private health sector. The inequities in distribution of health services among different social classes, therefore, remain a prominent characteristic of the health care system in Peru. Although improvements are occurring, as reflected in such measures as a declining infant mortality rate, this transitional country still has a long way to go to reach the majority of its population with scientific health service.

An Underdeveloped Country System—Ghana

Ghana is by no means the poorest country in Africa but, as a former British colony emancipated after World War II, it probably offers a fair illustration of the health care systems found generally in sub-Sahara Africa. Ghana is located on the northwest coast of the continent.

In terms of economic investment in health service, as in most African countries, this is quite low—an estimated 1.8 percent of the gross national product. A significant part of even this small slice of the Ghanaian economic pie comes from international donations, either through foreign governmental aid or religious missions. Domestically, the source of economic support is mainly private payments and central governmental revenues. Ninety percent of the 1970 population of 8.5 million depend for their scientific health services on resources supported essentially by government revenues, but use of public hospitals and health centers or even the facilities operated by religious missions usually requires payment of small private fees.

Traditional healers in the villages must also be paid privately. The 10 percent or smaller portion of the population who pay entirely for private medical care, combined with the other private expenditures, probably account for 40 to 50 percent of total monies going for health purposes. The balance, then, comes mainly from general revenues, with small fractions coming from private industry and philanthropy. No economic contribution is derived from insurance, social or voluntary.

The approximate distribution of economic support for health care in Ghana may be inferred from the mode of work of physicians. In 1970, there were 667 doctors in the nation, yielding a doctor-population ratio of 1:12,700. Of these, slightly over half were foreigners working either in missions or in the government service. The latter employs 369 (or 55 percent) of the doctors, although some of these engage in private practice when they are off duty. It is noteworthy that in 1961 the doctor-population ratio had been 1:18,000, so it has improved. The proportion of doctors in government service then, however, was 64 percent, so that the proportion practicing in the private sector has evidently risen.

The geographic distribution of doctors in Ghana is even more uneven than that in Peru. Of the available doctors, more than 50 percent are in the capital region in and around Accra, where under 10 percent of the population live. The balance of doctors must serve the remaining 90 percent of the population, meaning that for the majority the supply ratio is much poorer than 1:12,700. In the Upper Ghana region with nearly 900,000 people, for example, there are eight doctors, a ratio of fewer than 1:100,000.

The most numerous type of health manpower in Ghana is doubtless the traditional healer—witch doctors and village midwives—on whom the mass of the rural population must depend for most of their health care. Traditional healing in Ghana, unlike Asia, is based mostly on the invocation of supernatural spirits, rather than empirically accumulated remedies. Local healers tend to have great prestige, and the effectiveness of some of their ministrations may relate to the patient's confidence in them.

Probably because of the colonial medical service heritage, the supply of auxiliary health personnel, relative to physicians, is greater in Ghana than in Peru. In 1970 there were 7,350 nurses of all levels, the great majority being equivalent to the vocational nurse of the industrialized countries. Some 40 percent of the nurses are men, and they give a great deal of the primary care at rural health stations and health centers. In 1970, there were only forty-one trained dentists in all of Ghana, or a ratio of less than 1:200,000. Midwives, on the other hand, have been trained in relatively large numbers, there being 2,808 in 1970 or a ratio of about 1:3,000.

Health facilities are more numerous in Ghana than in most countries of black Africa but still are more meager than in the transitional countries. In 1971, there were 203 hospitals of all types (including small rural units) with 11,300 beds; this meant a ratio of 1.28 beds per 1,000 population. About 67 percent of these beds were in government structures, and the rest were in facilities operated by religious missions, commercial enterprises, private nonprofit bodies, or purely proprietary owners.

In contrast to Tanzania in southeast Africa or many Asian countries, health centers for ambulatory care are fewer in Ghana than are hospitals. In 1971, there were forty-nine health centers, each intended to serve 200,000 people, and twenty governmental health posts, each supposedly serving 15,000 people. An indeterminate number of small dispensaries are operated by local authorities and staffed by villagers with uncertain training.

The pattern of delivery of primary health care in Ghana is obviously dependent mainly on traditional healers and briefly trained nurses who staff the health centers or health posts. The physicians in government service have time to serve only a small portion of the patients seeking ambulatory care, so that they spend most of their time in supervising auxiliary personnel or in treating hospital bedpatients. Only a very small proportion of the doctors are specialists —probably less than 10 percent. Service from a specialist, for the vast majority of the population, requires being at a hospital, either as an inpatient or outpatient. Specialist care in a private office is accessible only to the small affluent fraction of people concentrated in the few main cities.

As in most impoverished tropical countries, the infectious and parasitic diseases are very prominent in Ghana, and yet organized preventive services have had only a slight impact on them. An infant mortality rate between 100 and 200 per 1,000 live births is due largely to water- or food-borne infections (gastroenteritis, dysentery, etc.), but most of the population must still depend on insanitary water supplies. Refrigeration of food is possible in only a handful of wealthy households. Preventive child and maternal health services are given in conjunction with medical care at health centers and health posts, but only a small fraction of the population have access to these units. Immunizations are provided for only a minority of the children, with the exception of smallpox vaccination, which was the subject of a centrally managed campaign launched in 1960 with the aid of the World Health Organization. A national campaign has also provided BCG vaccination against tuberculosis to 300,000 susceptible persons. Protein and calorie malnutrition in small children after weaning is a critical problem, but relatively little has been done in an organized way to deal with this.

Perhaps typical of the strategy in the underdeveloped countries of Africa is a demonstration project on rural health and family planning services in a group of villages around Danfa, a town close to Accra, the national capital. The project was launched by the University of Ghana Medical School, established in 1964, to provide a field training center for medical students. It is financed, however, by the United States Agency for International Development (USAID) and is operated in cooperation with the University of California at Los Angeles. The Danfa Project, by establishing comparison villages with different inputs of health services, is attempting to demonstrate the outcomes in death and sickness rates and other measurements of various sorts of modern preventive, family planning, and curative health services provided from health centers. Assuming it is found to be effective, whether this model of delivering health care, dependent as it is on substantial external funding, can be replicated later in other parts of Ghana remains to be seen.

The Ghanaian health services are, in the main, administered centrally; local government is weak and unimportant. Whatever regulation of personnel, facilities, or drugs is exercised comes from the national Ministry of Health. With a succession of military governments in Ghana over the last thirty years, democracy in the Western sense is virtually nonexistent, and appointments from the Minister of Health down are essentially on political grounds. Coordination of services is not a significant problem because there is no multiplicity of agencies; no major competing medical care program under social security agency control, such as in Peru, is found. Likewise, there is no rising wave of consumer demand for participation or control of health care policy, such as one sees in better educated populations. The voluntary agencies, mainly religious missions, are rather well integrated with the governmental services; the Ministry of Health looks upon mission hospitals or clinics as additional resources, relieving government of obligations to establish facilities in areas so served.

Health planning in Ghana has been all too typical of that in many underdeveloped countries—very ambitious on paper and feeble in accomplishment. This comment is based on information from Ghanaian sources. The former Director of Medical Services of Ghana writes in 1973:

> In 1963 a Planning Commission including two doctors was set up, and a comprehensive national development plan was written. This plan, which was not implemented, was very ambitious. It aimed to provide for very rapid development of hospital services and at the same time for expansion of promotive, protective, and preventive services—an almost impossible task. . . . After the coup of 1966 this plan was shelved. . . . (A new committee), reporting two years later stated that the emphasis should be on the promotive and the protective services . . . and training of health personnel. Nothing was done to implement this committee's report. In 1971 another committee was set up (for) devising a health-sector plan. . . . This committee reported towards the end of 1971 . . . when the Government which ordered it was overthrown by another military coup. . . . Thus the latest attempt to produce a health plan can be regarded as stillborn.

Effective planning of health services, especially in a very poor country, depends on willingness to harness all resources, both public and private, and on long-term government stability. It is clear that neither of these conditions is found in Ghana.

Priorities in Ghana would generally be stated by the national health officials as improved environmental sanitation, control of communicable diseases, and primary health care in the rural areas. In practice, the major share of resources is devoted to hospital services in the main cities and general personal health care to the affluent minority of families.

A Socialist System—The Soviet Union

Although many differences have developed among the world's fully socialist countries, we may take as illustrative the first one to launch an enduring socialist revolution: the Soviet Union. Even countries like the People's Republic of China, which have become quite different from the USSR in their political policies, still have a health service system with many similarities (in spite of some notable differences) to the Soviet model.

The economic support of Soviet health services is easy to describe, since it is so basically simple. With minor exceptions, the support is derived from the general revenues of the government which, in turn, come from the production of all commodities. Most of this (about 57 percent) comes from the national government budget, and nearly all of the balance from the earnings of local enterprises, collective farms, or other public bodies—equivalent in other societies to local units of government. Only a trivial percentage of the total expenditure for health service (perhaps 2 to 3 percent) comes from private payments for certain drugs, dental prostheses, or a very small amount of private care. Altogether about 4.0 percent (varying from 3.9 to 4.2 percent in recent years) of total Soviet national income (the Soviet economists do not make use of the gross national product concept in their calculations) is spent on health services. This is a much lower percentage, it will be recalled, than the comparable share of GNP in the United States or most other industrialized countries.

This largely unitary source of financing of health services in the Soviet Union today (public revenues) has been a product of sixty years of development since the 1917 Revolution. Private medical practice was never banned by law, and it did not die out until the public medical system was effectively built up. For the first twenty years after the Revolution, a social security program operated for the urban industrial workers, while a separate general revenue system supported health services for the rural population. Then the financing of these two large sectors was united in 1938 under a unified Ministry of Health.

The Soviet Constitution guarantees complete preventive and therapeutic health care to everyone as a public service. To accomplish this, great emphasis has been put on the training of health manpower. Medical schools were developed at most large provincial (*oblast*) hospitals and in all the main cities, turning out thousands of doctors at a rate much faster than the growth of population. Around 1937 all but a few medical schools (eighty one of them) were transferred from the universities under the Ministry of Education to the Ministry of Health, where their policies could be made more directly responsive to the health needs of the people. Great emphasis in the medical institutes, as the schools are now called, is put on preventive and social medicine, as well as on the everyday management of common ailments. The medical curriculum lasts six years after high school, as in Europe generally.

The numbers of doctors trained increased rapidly. The supply in Russia before the Revolution in 1913 was 0.14 per 1,000. By 1940, it had risen to 0.79 per 1,000 and in 1975 to 3.25 per 1,000, or a ratio to population of 1:308. This is about twice the proportion found in the United States. It must be realized, however, that medicine in the Soviet Union is considered a very stressful occupation, so that the normal working day is only six hours, much shorter than in America or most other countries. On the other hand, there are thousands of *feldshers*, with a wide scope of responsibilities similar to those of the American nurse practitioner, although with the abundance of doctors *feldshers* are being withdrawn from primary care. There are also thousands of nurses, more numerous than doctors, plus midwives and many other health workers. Laboratory technicians and clerical personnel, however, are relatively fewer than in the United States, since less emphasis is put on refinements in diagnostic technology, and the administrative tasks are much fewer. The majority of Soviet physicians, as well as other health workers, are women.

Specialization in medicine has been growing as in the welfare state health systems but, at about 40 percent of the total doctors, is not as great as in the United States. Much emphasis is placed on child health care, so that pediatricians are regarded as general practitioners for children rather than as specialists. Medical students follow one of three basic tracks: general therapeutics, pediatrics, and hygiene. After completion of training, all must spend three years in a rural or other underserved location. Following this they may move back to a city, if they wish, although larger salaries are offered to induce them to stay on. Later they may undertake postgraduate study at designated institutes to prepare for a specialty.

Most dental care is given by relatively briefly trained dental doctors who do simple prophylaxes, fillings, dental health education, and so on. They work under the direction of stomatologists, who are physicians specializing in diseases of the mouth, in the same sense that ophthalmologists are specialists for the eye.

Altogether, the Soviet Union had in 1971 about 698,000 doctors, 2,195,000 middle-range personnel (*feldshers*, nurses, technicians, etc.), and other health workers adding up to 5.6 percent of the total work force. Although, as we have noted, the composition of health manpower differs, this compares very closely to the total proportion in the United States, which in 1971 for its working population of about 80 million had 4.4 million health personnel, constituting 5.5 percent of the total work force. Yet, these American health manpower, plus the expenses of drugs, construction, research, and so on absorb over 8 percent of the United States GNP, compared with 4 percent of national income for comparable purposes in the USSR.

All Soviet doctors work on salaries that are scaled according to their training, skill, seniority, and responsibility. Salaries are not so high as in capitalist countries, being comparable to those of school teachers or skilled manual workers. However, physicians command as much prestige as elsewhere, and there are two or three applications for every medical school opening. Except in some very thinly settled rural districts, all doctors work along with nurses and other allied personnel in teams at health centers, polyclinics, or hospitals.

All the health facilities are owned and operated by the central Ministry of Health although their management is delegated in a pyramidal structure to the USSR's fifteen constituent republics, then to the provinces (*oblast*), regions (*rayon*), and to neighborhoods (*uchastok*) at the most local level. Some rest homes are administered by labor unions, but all health facilities are government property. Principles of regionalization are applied, with the management of each hospital coming under the supervision of the facility at the next higher echelon. Patients are referred to the level of hospital proper for their condition, and ambulances for transport are attached to each institution. The supply of hospital beds is high, at over 11 per 1,000, and the great majority of these beds are for general illness.

The hospital administration consists of a director, generally a physician who also does some clinical work, aided by an administrative deputy. There is no board of directors in the Western European or American sense, except that a committee of hospital employees is usually advisory to the director. The medical staff, being entirely salaried and organized in a systematic framework, is under continuous peer review, rather than being subject to a post hoc review based on a study of records. Hospital outpatient departments offer ambulatory specialist services, although most such services are given at polyclinics. Many hospitals conduct educational programs for middle-range personnel, as well as for doctors. Research, on the other hand, is conducted in separate institutes, some of which may be affiliated with hospitals; research is not typically linked to teaching, as in the United States.

Primary care of the general population is given at polyclinics in the cities or at health centers in rural areas, which still contain a relatively high 42 percent of the Soviet population. The pattern of delivery is defined as "districting," in the sense that a general adult doctor or therapeutist is responsible for primary care of about 2,000 people in a geographic district. Likewise, a pediatrician is responsible for 1,000 children in a designated area. If a patient is dissatisfied with the doctor serving his or her district, he can apply for transfer to another doctor, although this is said to happen seldom. The therapeutist and pediatrician both try to spend a part of each day on home calls, which are considered important to acquaint the doctor with each family's living conditions. In addition, these primary care doctors do all the personal preventive service, including health education at an expected rate of a half hour per day.

"Dispensarization" is an important feature of Soviet preventive health services. All persons considered especially vulnerable—not only small children and pregnant women, but older persons with chronic illness, workers exposed to certain hazards, adolescents, and others—are called back to the polyclinic or health center for periodic checkups. There are also clinics at the larger factories, where such checkups are done, and general care of chronic disease and simple primary care for minor illness or injuries are provided as well.

Mental health services seem to receive less emphasis in the Soviet health system than in other industrialized countries. There are some special psychiatric clinics in the main cities, but not many. Mental hospital beds constitute only about 10 percent of the total, or about one bed per 1,000. Therapy for mental disorder emphasizes physical modalities and group occupational activities.

The preventive health services, as we have said, are integrated closely with the therapeutic services on the level of personal health care. There are, however, sanitary-epidemiological or "sanepid" stations concerned largely with environmental sanitation and control of the communicable diseases, including certain mass campaigns of immunization or case detection. Sometimes the sanepid stations may be under the administration of the nearby hospital, but in the large cities, they are separate and report directly to the health department authority of the *oblast*. Routine child and maternal health services are given at the polyclinics by the same child or adult doctor who serves the family generally, although special hours of the week may be scheduled for these preventive services. Family planning advice is offered on request, and abortions are legal for any psychosocial or medical reason. At this time, multiphasic screening for hidden disease is not being promoted in the USSR, although the periodic dispensarization procedure may detect hypertension, diabetes, or some other chronic disorder.

Health care regulation is basically built into the whole Soviet health system, so that it does not require much special attention. All graduates of Soviet training institutes are authorized to work, as long as they have passed their schools' examinations. Hospitals and health centers, being owned and controlled by the Ministry of Health, are periodically inspected by ministerial officials. If there have been problems, a special investigation may be made. Day-to-day medical performance is under ongoing surveillance, so that subsequent medical audits are not performed, and one does not hear of any malpractice litigation. Complaints of patients are taken to the health facility administrator for redress or, if serious, to the local political party unit. A doctor or other health worker considered culpable may be transferred or penalized in some way.

Drug control is not difficult because all drug manufacturing is under the direction of the Ministry of Health. Only one or two products of each pharmacological action are manufactured in government factories, or sometimes imported. Drugs are distributed by the Ministry of Health to all hospitals and polyclinics, as well as to local government-operated pharmacies. At these pharmacies, anyone may purchase certain nonprescribed or ameliorative drugs (such as sleeping pills, vitamins, aspirin, cough syrups, etc.) for which he must pay, but drugs essential for treatment (such as antibiotics, insulin, digitalis, etc.) are either dispensed at the polyclinic or hospital or may be obtained at a pharmacy without charge.

The administrative structure of the Soviet health services is maintained through a surprisingly simple hierarchical network of authority emanating from the national Ministry of Health in Moscow outward to the fifteen republic ministries, then to health departments in the provinces or *oblasts*. These health departments are responsible for *all* health services—preventive and therapeutic, ambulatory and hospital, general and special—in their territory. Each *oblast* is further subdivided into regions or *rayons,* and these into neighborhoods or *uchastocks.* As noted above, the hospital is regarded not solely as a health care facility for the seriously sick but as an administrative center for supervising the ambulatory care facilities peripheral to it and sometimes for supervising the sanepid stations.

The Ministry of Health is responsible not only for all personal and environmental health services but for health manpower education as well. Through its Academy of Medical Sciences, which supervises hundreds of specialized scientific institutes, it supervises research as well, so that investigative efforts will be focused on problems deemed important for the health care system. The manufacture of drugs, supplies, and medical equipment also comes under ministry direction. Health services in the factories and schools are part of the same system, although their financial support may come from other sources.

The top official, the Minister of Health, is invariably a doctor who has been chosen by the ruling Communist Party and is a member of the Council of Ministers. This official and his or her counterpart in each republic (this minister is often a woman) is appointed with obvious consideration of political reliability first and technical competence second. Since the whole system is unified, there are no special problems of coordinating multiple agencies. Consumerism is expressed through various organizations of labor unions, women, farmers, youth, and so on at the local level, who express their views to the local political party units. Paperwork in the Soviet health system is scanty because the program operates under well-understood rules and does not require the variety of administrative procedures for special population groups or special diseases or services that one sees in the United States, Western Europe or elsewhere.

Comprehensive planning plays a central part in the Soviet health system. Starting from a national planning institute (Semashko) in Moscow, standards or norms are established for all types of health personnel and facilities in large cities, intermediate towns, and rural areas. These norms are determined through empirical studies of service utilization carried out periodically, with the findings modified by theoretical considerations, such as the extent of nonsymptomatic disease and projections of changes in the disease prevalence or in medical potentialities in the future. Consideration must also be given to the expected productivity of doctors (e.g., the number of patients who can be reasonably served per hour) and others. The norms so derived are changed from time to time with the changing availability of doctors and allied health personnel, transportation improvements, and so on.

The norms are the basis for preparation of plans of work and budgets at the local level that are submitted to higher echelons for review, and eventually funds are allocated from the central Ministry of Health to all local units. (This process differs in the People's Republic of China, where much greater latitude is exercised at the local level. This policy of local self-reliance has inspired Chinese health personnel and others to work very hard, but it means, of course, great variation in the standards of health service achieved in different localities.) Every five years, a new health plan setting goals for the coming period is made in the Soviet Union. At the central level, an agency called GOSPLAN decides on the overall allocation of funds to the health services, compared with housing, education, military purposes, steel production, and so on. (See earlier discussion on page 193.) It is this distributional decision that ultimately determines the 4.0 percent of national income currently going to the health sector in the USSR, which, in turn, affects the salaries that may be paid to doctors, the staffing of hospitals or polyclinics, and so on.

Priorities in the Soviet health system appear to be highest for children and for industrial workers. Preventive service in general is also emphasized in comparison with policies of other industrialized countries. The pervasive priority, one might say, is on quantity of health care more than quality. The foremost goal has been to achieve delivery of at least a modest level of comprehensive health care to the total far-flung Soviet population, rather than to attain a technologically superior level of services that would only reach a small fraction of people.

By free enterprise or even welfare state criteria, the Soviet health system would be considered highly regimented. Medical service is not a private independent enterprise, every health worker is part of an organized team, there is little free choice of doctor or other health provider. Yet, from the viewpoint of the Soviet citizen, the system provides everyone with virtually free and comprehensive health service. Compared with other industrialized countries, the wages of the average Soviet worker, manual or white-collar, are relatively low, but he has no problem in paying for health care and it is readily accessible at any time. The lack or very limited degree of freedom of choice of doctor does not seem to bother him, and foreign observers have been generally impressed with the high level of satisfaction of the Soviet people with their health care system.

Main Trends

With such a great variety of health care systems in the world and with diverse trends in each of them, perhaps it is foolhardy to attempt a summary of the main trends. Still, if one is willing to accept some oversimplifications and to recognize that there are exceptions, sometimes important ones, to every generalization, perhaps a number of general trends in health service can be identified in the many nations of the world. Although each country is undergoing changes in ways that correspond to its political, economic, and sociocultural setting, the following broad trends can be observed:

1. Economic support for health services is, on the whole, becoming more collectivized. Private payments are playing a lesser relative role, whereas insurance—mainly social rather than voluntary—and general revenues are playing an enlarging role. Along with this, a slowly increasing share of national GNP is being devoted to health purposes.

2. The supply of doctors relative to population in all countries is increasing. In the less developed countries, specialization is also growing, but in the more industrialized countries a reaction against excessive specialization has set in, and the general medical practitioner is being strengthened both in quality and numbers.

3. The range of other allied health personnel, either working with the doctor or doing special tasks independently, is widening and their supply (ratio to population) is also increasing. For primary health care in the less developed countries, many forms of doctor substitute are being produced in relatively short periods, and in some industrialized countries such personnel are also being trained for underserved areas.

4. Health facilities are increasing in number and in their technical capabilities. More general hospital beds in relation to population are being constructed in the developing countries, although in several affluent countries there is a sense that an adequate or even excessive supply has been built. In all types of country, more facilities are also being constructed for provision of ambulatory health services, curative and preventive, in organized frameworks. The sponsorship of both hospitals and ambulatory care health centers is being increasingly vested in government bodies. Even private individual doctors are teaming up in group practice clinics with mounting frequency.

5. The patterns for delivery of all levels of medical care are becoming increasingly systematized. Primary and ambulatory care is more often being provided by teams in health centers of various sorts. Services in hospitals are increasingly being furnished by salaried specialists in organized frameworks. In general, the remuneration of doctors by fees for each unit of service is gradually being replaced by payment for the doctor's time, through salaries—usually rather high.

6. The value of preventive services is becoming increasingly appreciated everywhere. This applies not only to the communicable, nutritional, or traumatic diseases but also to the metabolic or degenerative disorders, the prevention of which depends in large part on modification of personal behavior. The line between prevention and treatment is becoming steadily more blurred, so that delivery of personal preventive services is becoming more and more integrated with delivery of the treatment services. Environmental health services, on the other

hand, are often becoming integrated with general environmental control measures that are not necessarily linked to the health sector.

7. Because of the rising utilization and over-all cost of health services everywhere (or the rising share of national GNP being allocated to health), greater attention is being given to regulation of these expenditures. Likewise, because of the increasing complexities of science, greater public concern is being shown for surveillance over the quality of the services provided. No longer is the doctor or hospital regarded as beyond the challenge of the humble patient. All sorts of procedures, governmental and voluntary, are being developed to exercise controls over the costs and quality of health care.

8. To cope with the mounting complexities of all the organized settings developed for providing different types of health service, efforts are being made everywhere to design more effective administration of total health care systems. To do this, government is playing an increasing supervisory role, but the voluntary or private sector is also becoming more systematized. The voice of the consumer in relation to the provider of health service is becoming stronger. Coordination of multiple health agencies, which have arisen historically, is being promoted, with a movement toward more integrated or even unitary systems. To achieve equity for people at all geographic locations, regionalized networks of authority are being established so that patients may be readily referred from peripheral to central facilities, and special skills may be extended from the center peripherally. Systematic national health planning is becoming accepted everywhere as necessary.

All eight of these trends tend to reinforce one another. There are, of course, exceptions in one or another country from time to time, when particular political or economic circumstances may promote changes in the direction of individualistic rather than social concepts in health care. The long-term pressure of the popular will, however, is toward achieving the goal spelled out in the United Nations Universal Declaration of Human Rights in 1948, which states:

> Everyone has the right to a standard of living adequate for health and well-being of himself and of his family, including . . . medical care . . . and the right to security in the event of sickness.

Probably no nation has yet reached this health ideal, but a study of the world makes clear that, at different paces and along different paths, all countries are moving toward it. In human terms, this is coming to mean the development of systems of health care in which the priorities will ultimately be based not on individual resources but on the optimal social good.

Readings

Anderson, Odin W., *The Uneasy Equilibrium*, New Haven: College and University Press, 1968.

Brown, R. G. S., *The Changing National Health Service*, Boston: Routledge and Kegan Paul, 1973.

Douglas-Wilson, I. and Gordon MacLachlen (eds.), *Health Service Prospects: An International Survey*, London: The Lancet, 1973.

Dwivedi, J. K., "Medical Care in India," *World Hospitals, 3*:40-45 (1967).

Evang, Karl, D. S. Murray, and W. J. Lear, *Medical Care and Family Security: Norway, England, USA*, Englewood Cliffs, N.J.: Prentice-Hall, 1963.

Evang, Karl, *The Health Services of Norway*, Oslo: Hammerstad Boktrgkkeri, 1969.

Falk, I. S., "Medical Care in the U.S.A.: 1932-1972," *Health and Society, 51*: 1-32 (Winter 1973).

Field, Mark G., *Soviet Socialized Medicine: An Introduction*, New York: Free Press, 1967.

Fry, John, *Medicine in Three Societies: A Comparison of Medical Care in the USSR, USA, and UK*, New York: American Elsevier Co., 1970.

Goodman, Neville M., *International Medical Organizations and Their Work*, 2nd ed., Edinburgh: Churchill Livingstone, 1971.

Grushka, T. (ed.), *Health Services in Israel*, Jerusalem: Ministry of Health, 1968.

Hensey, Brendan, *The Health Services of Ireland*, Dublin: Institute of Public Administration, 1972.

Hyde, Gordon, *The Soviet Health Service: A Historical and Comparative Analysis*, London: Lawrence & Wishart, 1974.

Ingman, Stan R. and Anthony E. Thomas (eds.), *Topias and Utopias in Health: Policy Studies*, The Hague: Mouton Publishers, 1974.

Japanese Ministry of Health & Welfare, *Health Services in Japan*, Tokyo, 1974.

Kacprzak, M. and B. Kozusznik, *Health Care in Poland*, Warsaw: Polonia Publishing House, 1963.

Kohn, Robert and Susan Radius, "Two Roads to Health Care: U.S. and Canadian Policies 1945-1975," *Medical Care, 12*:189-201 (March 1974).

Lalonde, M., *A New Perspective on Health of Canadians*, Ottawa: Department of National Health & Welfare, 1974.

Lindsey, Almont, *Socialized Medicine in England and Wales: The National Health Service 1948-1961*, Chapel Hill: University of North Carolina Press, 1962.

Mahmud, Siraj-ul-Haq, "Health Services in Pakistan," *World Hospitals, 6*:16-25 (1970).

Margan, Ivo, "The Yugoslav Health System," *World Hospitals, 6*:76-79 (April 1970).

Meade, T. W., "Medicine in India," *The Lancet*, 27 June 1970, pp. 1381-1383.

Mechanic, David, "The English National Health Service: Some Comparisons with the United States," *Journal of Health and Social Behavior, 12*:18-29 (March 1971).

——, "Health Status and Medical Care in the Republic of South Africa," in *Politics, Medicine, and Social Science,* New York: John Wiley, 1974, pp. 21-35.

Mikho, Emanuel, "Health Services in Iraq and the Problems and Factors Affecting Their Provision," *World Hospitals, 8*:288-294 (1972).

Myrdal, Gunnar, *Beyond the Welfare State,* New Haven: Yale University Press, 1960.

Querido, A., *The Development of Socio-Medical Care in the Netherlands,* London: Routledge and Kegan Paul, 1968.

Quinn, Joseph R. (ed.), *Medicine and Public Health in the People's Republic of China,* Washington, D.C.: U.S. Dept. of Health, Education, and Welfare, 1972.

Roemer, Milton I., *Medical Care in Latin America,* Washington, D.C.: Pan American Union, 1963.

——, *Cuban Health Services and Resources,* Washington, D.C.: Pan American Health Organization, 1976.

Sai, F. T. et al., "The Danfa/Ghana Comprehensive Rural Health and Family Planning Project—A Community Approach," *Ghana Medical Journal, 11*: 9-17 (1972).

Schram, Ralph, *A History of Nigerian Health Services,* New York: Holmes and Meier, 1972.

Selby, Philip, *Health in 1980-1990,* Basel: S. Karger, 1974.

Sidel, Victor W. and Ruth Sidel, *Serve the People: Observations on Medicine in the People's Republic of China,* New York: Josiah Macy Jr. Foundation, 1973.

Sigerist, Henry E., *Medicine and Health in the Soviet Union,* New York: Citadel Press, 1947.

Singh, K., "An Outline of the Medical Services in Malaysia," *Medical Journal of Malaya, 25*:79-82 (1970).

Titmuss, R. M. and B. Abel-Smith, *The Health Services of Tanganyika,* London: Pitman, 1964.

Vukmanovic, C., "Decentralized Socialism: Medical Care in Yugoslavia," *International Journal of Health Services, 2*:35-44 (1972).

Winter, Kurt (ed.), *Public Health in the German Democratic Republic,* Berlin: Post-graduate Medical School of the German Democratic Republic, c. 1970.

Woodruff, A. W., "Medicine in Burma Today," *British Medical Journal, 3*:551-554 (1967).

World Health Organization, Regional Office for Europe, *Health Services in Europe,* Copenhagen, WHO, 1965.

INDEX

A

Abortion, 11, 159, 229
Access to health care, 114, 204, 206
Accreditation associations, 168 (*see
    also* Licensure; Specialty Boards)
Acupuncture, 8, 71, 74, 87, 120
Advertising, 65, 177
Aerial medical services, 130
Aesculapius, 52, 90
Afghanistan, 16
Africa, 16-17, 27, 44, 127, 134, 151,
    155, 159 (*see also individual
    countries*)
    colonial influence on health care
        in, 4, 54-55
    health care administration, 189
    health care planning, 196-198
    health workers, 76, 77, 80, 84, 85,
        86
    hospitals, 91, 92, 94, 100
    medical education, 56-57, 64
    regionalization of care, 106
    specialists, 122
    traditional healers, 71, 73
African sleeping sickness, 145
Aged, health care of, 12, 46, 96, 97,
    98, 129, 132-134 (*see also*
    Medicare)
Agricultural health hazards, 143
Air pollution, 143
Alcoholism, 131, 144, 160
Ambulatory care (*see also* Hospital
    outpatient departments;
    Polyclinics)

[Ambulatory care]
    facilities for, 100, 103, 106, 109,
        232
    India, 198
    Peru, 220
    Soviet Union, 99
    transitional countries, 18
    underdeveloped countries, 16
    U.S., 27, 55
American Hospital Association, 34
American Indians, 45, 93
American Medical Association, 59, 65-
    66, 121, 166, 168
American Pharmaceutical Association,
    168
American Public Health Association,
    185
American Revolution
    influence on health care system, 2
American Society of Clinical Patholo-
    gists, 167
Angola, 196
Apothecary, 50, 53, 80
Argentina, 56, 62
Artisans' guilds, 33
Asia, 16, 44, 64, 122, 134, 151, 155
    (*see also* Colonialism *and the
    individual countries*)
    herbalists in, 110
    hospitals of, 91, 106
Association of American Medical
    Colleges, 168
Audiologists, 50, 82, 154

237

H